£3.99

HOMEOPATHY
FOR EMOTIONAL HEALTH

Rima Handley was born and educated in Blackpool, then went to Oxford University where she studied medieval English language and literature. She taught medieval literature at the universities of London and Newcastle upon Tyne for several years, then gave up the academic life to train and practise first as a homoeopath and subsequently as a psychotherapist. She now combines the practice of both psychotherapy and homoeopathy.

She was co-founder of the Northern College of Homeopathic Medicine, one of the first homoeopathic training colleges to be established in the UK, and still takes an active part in the running of the College. She has written three other books about homoeopathy: *A Homeopathic Love Story*, a biography of the founder of homoeopathy, Samuel Hahnemann and his wife Melanie, the first woman homoeopath (published by North Atlantic Books in 1990); *Homoeopathy for Women* (published by Thorsons, 1993); and *In Search of the Later Hahnemann* (published by Beaconsfield Press, 1995). She practises in Newcastle and in Thirsk, North Yorkshire.

HOMOEOPATHY FOR EMOTIONAL HEALTH

Rima Handley

Thorsons
An Imprint of HarperCollinsPublishers

Thorsons
An Imprint of HarperCollins*Publishers*
77–85 Fulham Palace Road,
Hammersmith, London W6 8JB
1160 Battery Street,
San Francisco, California 94111-1213

Published by Thorsons 1995

1 3 5 7 9 10 8 6 4 2

© Rima Handley 1995

Rima Handley asserts the moral right to
be identified as the author of this work

A catalogue record for this book
is available from the British Library

ISBN 0 7225 2965 1

Printed in Great Britain by
HarperCollinsManufacturing Glasgow

Dedicated to Simone

CONTENTS

PART THREE
Materia Medica

ACKNOWLEDGEMENTS

Many people have helped me write this book: some by reading it while it was in progress and encouraging me, offering support and suggestions; others by doing things for me which freed me to write when I could; yet others merely by being there. I'd like to thank them all very warmly:

Naona Beecher-Moore, Alan Brice, Carol Cartridge, Don Cartridge, Diana Clarke, Christine Conyers, Connie Driver, Caroline Grist, Inca, Glynis Ingram, Mandy Little, Rasta, Lindsay River, Simone Silverpath, Barbara Vesey and all my colleagues, students, patients and clients. In compiling the *Materia Medica* pictures I have made use of the published *Materia Medica* of Catherine Coulter, Douglas Gibson, Jacques Jouanny and Robin Murphy, as well as unpublished material derived from the lectures of George Vithoulkas. I'd also like to acknowledge my general debt to all homoeopaths living and dead, particularly to Samuel Hahnemann.

Note to the Reader

Properly used, homoeopathic remedies are safe and without side-effects. If in doubt consult a qualified practitioner. Neither the publishers nor the author accepts any responsibility for any effects that may arise from giving or taking any remedy included in this book.

PREFACE

Calling a book *Homoeopathy for Emotional Health* may seem a rather strange thing to do, may be thought to suggest from the beginning that emotions can or should be treated, even cured, with homoeopathy. From the outset I want to dispel this idea. In Britain, at any rate, we are only just beginning to get used to the idea of expressing emotions, abandoning the stiff upper lip (the legacy of centuries of repression and cold weather): it would be a terrible pity if we started 'curing' this self-expression now.

No. What this book is about is how to use homoeopathy to help balance your emotions and feel better for it. It is *imbalance* of the emotions that causes all the trouble, not having them or expressing them. Such an imbalance springs from many sources: genetic, environmental, spiritual, physical, cultural. Homoeopathy is a system of medicine that works by trying to bring about a balanced relationship between all these different parts of ourselves.

How homoeopathy does this is still something of a mystery, though there are some theories about it which we will look at in this book. That it does so is beyond question: many thousands of satisfied patients will testify to the difference homoeopathic treatment has made to their lives, how it has helped them feel better, feel more in tune with themselves, and how, specifically, it has relieved them of conditions such as depression, anxiety and sleeplessness as well as a host of physical complaints that are not the particular province of this book.

One patient has said:

> I didn't really go to the homoeopath because I was depressed.
> I went because I had pains in my chest. Actually I didn't even
> tell her I'd been depressed for years because I'd sort of got
> used to it. I'd been taking anti-depressants for a long time and
> it was better than it had been and I thought that was what I
> was stuck with for the rest of my life. After a few weeks,
> though, I began to notice how much happier I felt, and I
> haven't been really depressed since.

Homoeopathy is one of the safest and most effective forms of
medicine that has ever been discovered. If you have already used it
for first-aid treatments you will know the amazing effect that *Arnica*
has on an injury, *Nux vomica* on a stomach upset or *Chamomilla* on
the mood of a screaming child. Its usefulness in simple cases is well
known. Nowadays large pharmacies are stocking the remedies and
encouraging people to use them on their own initiative to cure
minor ailments. You need very little knowledge to make your own
successful homoeopathic first-aid prescriptions.

However, homoeopathy is not just a first-aid medicine, it is also a
sophisticated healing system capable of addressing complex conditions of health and what is known as 'dis-ease'. What is used safely
and effectively in the home can also be used to greater effect under
the guidance of a trained homoeopath.

This book will explain clearly the principles and philosophy of
homoeopathy (so different from those of orthodox medicine), offer
a simple explanation of how homoeopathy works and how you can
use it to improve the emotional health of yourself and your family,
and will provide you with some information about how modern
homoeopaths prescribe.

Homoeopathy for Emotional Health is also intended to give you an
overview and a fuller understanding of how homoeopathy may be
used to treat more complex states of health, states that you will not
want to treat yourself but which you may be interested to find are
treatable by professional homoeopaths. Hence this book will talk
about the homoeopathic treatment of a whole range of illness, from
transient sleeplessness to schizophrenia.

There are nearly 3,000 remedies available for use in homoeopathy, and this can often seem daunting to the beginner. In this book I have chosen to talk about the use of a very small selection of commonly used and easily available remedies, so that it is possible for you to begin to use homoeopathy in a small way without being baffled by a mass of detail. If you are not successful in treating whatever you are trying to treat with the remedies specified in this book, don't give up, either go to a professional homoeopath and give him or her the job of discovering the less common remedy which the condition may need, or take your own studies further by going on a course at one of the Colleges listed in Appendix Two.

Interest in homoeopathy and other forms of alternative medicine has become great over the last few years, and more and more people are using it with success. It is important to get to know something about this form of medicine so that you can learn how it may benefit you. Homoeopathy is a very safe form of medicine: it uses remedies made from animal, vegetable and mineral substances prepared in such a way that they are powerful without being toxic. Even if, for example, a child were to swallow a bottle full of homoeopathic tablets, there would be no ill-effects.

The purpose of this book is twofold. First to make plain the principles and scope of homoeopathy in the treatment of emotional disturbance, and secondly to explain how you can treat acute conditions yourself. Obviously you should consult a professional homoeopath when your problem is not a temporary one. Successfully prescribing remedies for your own acute and mild conditions can, however, give you a sense of control and an appreciation of the possibilities for cure within homoeopathy. You can then go and get more experienced help for other more long-standing conditions.

You can discover the whereabouts of the trained homoeopaths in your area by writing to the Society of Homoeopaths for a list of registered homoeopaths or by contacting the homoeopathic training college nearest you. See Appendix Two for these addresses.

PART ONE

Homoeopathy and the Emotions

Chapter One

———

EMOTIONS, MIND, BODY AND SPIRIT

What are emotions? This may seem a silly question. Emotions are what we feel: happy, sad, angry, jealous, cross, content, anxious, fed up. Actually they can be quite transitory things: we can feel happy one minute, sad the next, depending on what is happening in our lives.

Emotional characteristics are like physical characteristics. We are born with the predisposition to develop a certain type of temperament just as we are born with a predisposition to develop a certain shape of nose. Some babies are smiling and relaxed from the moment of birth, others are squealing and shrieking, others are restless and crying. Our emotions are just as natural a part of us as our physical selves.

Just as our physical health is affected first by the genetic pattern at birth, then by chance infections, accidents, events, so our original genetically predetermined mode of emotional expression is influenced and moulded by circumstances: birth experience, upbringing, environment, chance events and our response to those events – nature and nurture shape our feelings and the way we express them.

One person may be born with a predisposition to chest complaints but grow out of them or, by moving to a less damp area of the country reduce his susceptibility to them; another may be born healthy and then be exposed to asbestos or gas and acquire a susceptibility to chest complaints. Likewise, someone might be born with a discontented disposition but be gifted with happy, placid parents whose attentions will modify this disposition; another child may be born with a happy, contented disposition but then be exposed to such trauma early in life that she becomes more melancholy: someone badly affected by war, for instance, or abuse or illness in the family.

We can acquire emotional dispositions in the same way we can acquire physical ones. And we can also look after our emotional selves and tendencies in the same way we do our physical ones. Emotional and physical are part of the same whole, not in any way separate.

This fact is increasingly recognized these days, even though we still often speak as if emotions are something different from, separate from the body. We acknowledge, for instance, that anxiety 'causes' headaches or gastric problems, that blocks in the expression of emotion may be implicated in the development of diseases such as cancer or rheumatoid arthritis. We also, on the other hand, describe some apparently emotional illnesses or problems as originating in physical disturbances: well-known examples are the emotional imbalances suffered by many women pre-menstrually, menopausally and during and after childbirth, said to be 'caused' by the variation in hormone levels. Adolescent boys and middle-aged men are similarly obviously affected emotionally by changes in their hormones. Imbalance in the output of the thyroid gland may also lead to emotional disturbances such as irritability, palpitations and panic attacks.

However, in reality it is incorrect to regard either emotional or physical spheres as the cause or origin of problems in the other. What is happening is that there is a disturbance in the whole energy or vitality of the person, an attack on what modern medicine limitingly calls the immune and defence system, which more traditional medicine variously calls the spirit, the vital force, or the vital principle.

When a person's vitality is affected, the consequent expression of dis-ease takes place on any level where that individual is susceptible to illness. It is important to recognize that this is the understanding of disease that underlies homoeopathy. This is why the homoeopath addresses the vitality of the whole person, not just the troublesome symptoms. If the disturbance in the vitality can be balanced then the disease will not need to express itself at all.

It may be helpful to use the analogy of the effects of 'stress', the modern explanation for almost all ills. 'Stress' expresses itself in various ways: physically, mentally or emotionally, according to the susceptibility of the person. Stress does not come about simply from working hard or from having a lot of difficulties to deal with: some people even thrive on this. Stress occurs when we have more demands made on us than we are able to cope with. And what this amounts to can vary from person to person, from time to time. Stress can cause a number of symptoms, whether these are predominantly physical – such as flushing, sweating, shallow breathing, chest pains, palpitations, headaches and backaches, vomiting and diarrhoea, constipation, fatigue, loss of appetite, irritable colon, dizziness, agitation, or shakiness – or predominantly psychological: sleep disturbances, panicky feelings, depression, irritability, worry, difficulty concentrating, forgetfulness, difficulty making decisions. In the same way, when a person's vitality is affected a variety of symptoms may arise, depending on that person's individual susceptibilities.

It is really neither the emotional nor the physical sphere which is the cause of these symptoms, but a disturbance in the whole body, expressed in particular ways by particular people. Some people *somatize*, that is, represent the disturbed state of their vitality in their bodies first; others express it through emotional distress; still others find that their intellectual functions – intelligence, memory and such things – are the first to break down.

Nowadays there is more and more evidence of a complex emotional/physiological feedback system in our bodies which is especially apparent in dis-eases such as cancer, rheumatoid arthritis, ME – in fact any of the auto-immune diseases. The 'new' science of psycho-neuro-immunology is proving what traditional medicine has always known: it is not enough to talk about emotions influencing the physical being or vice versa, each is an intrinsic part of the other.

Even so we are a long way from understanding this process in a truly holistic way, as the expression of a disorder in the body's energy field (vital force or spirit according to different models) manifested in either the emotional, physical or intellectual sphere, or in all three.

Traditional medicines have always recognized and worked with these intricate and implicit connections between mind, emotions and body. The more we learn, the more it is apparent that the modern Western medical way of thinking of the body and mind as distinct from each other – current only since the eighteenth century and Descartes' influential analysis of the body as a machine guided by the brain – is insufficient to explain the workings of the human organism. Neither mind nor matter is superior.

Fortunately homoeopathy, though emerging at the same time as modern Western medicine, developed along different lines and was from the beginning based on the concept of the co-existence of emotional and physical states: the way of prescribing homoeopathic remedies is based on approaching body and mind as a whole. The founder of homoeopathy, Samuel Hahnemann, wrote that 'there are no such things as diseases, there are only sick people', by which he meant that diseases are not separate entities but are conditioned and affected by the people in whom they occur. It is the *person*, *not* the disease, which is the object of homoeopathic cure. This is the cardinal principle of homoeopathic prescribing.

The homoeopath, therefore, looks at all the expressions of imbalance in a person, wherever these expressions are located: body, mind or emotions, and tries to select a remedy based on as whole a picture of all these signs of disorder as possible.

This brings us to the tricky question: How does homoeopathy work?

Chapter Two

HOW DOES
HOMOEOPATHY WORK?

A homoeopathic remedy works by raising the level of functioning of the immune system (vital force), so that it may respond to the appearance of any illness in a person, whatever form that illness takes. This increase in functioning is achieved by giving to the sick person minute doses of substances which would be capable (given in larger doses) of producing in a healthy person a symptom picture similar to that manifested by the sick person in illness.

A 'symptom picture' is a sort of overview of the person representing all of the symptoms and conditions, emotional and physical, which are expressive of the state of the person's health or ill-health at the time. The symptom picture can emerge as a result of illness or it can be produced artificially, by a drug or other toxic substance.

A homoeopathic remedy artificially emphasizes the sick person's symptoms, as it were increasing them slightly, bringing them out more clearly, in order to galvanize the body's self-healing system into action. Under the pressure of being given a mild further disease, similar to the one it already has, the human organism responds by throwing off both the original and the artificially-added disease. This, at least, was how Samuel Hahnemann, the eighteenth-century founder of homoeopathy, originally conceptualized what was happening. This is a process not unlike the one we are familiar with in vaccination, whereby immune system functioning is increased with respect to a particular disease. A homoeopathic remedy, on the other hand, produces a more general increase in immune system functioning so that a wider range of disease manifestations may be met by the revitalized immune system. In vaccination there are dangers from introducing a crude disease product into the body: these are avoided in homoeopathy by the use of highly diluted substances as remedies.

It is important to understand that these remedies are indeed very highly diluted. When Samuel Hahnemann first started working with homoeopathy he at first gave crude doses, as he was accustomed to doing in the orthodox medicine he had previously practised. However, since he was following the principle of similars, he found that these recreated the symptoms of the patient too strongly and so, over a number of years, he developed a method of diluting the strength of the remedies to make them less toxic (though no less powerful).

So, to look at the practical application of the idea of a symptom picture, if a person were, for instance, to complain of lying awake at night, unable to sleep for thinking about the day's events, was generally excitable, perhaps even having palpitations, she would be showing a symptom picture resembling what happens when a person drinks too much coffee. The remedy *Coffea* (prepared from highly diluted coffee), then, would probably be the one showing the most similar symptom picture to what the patient was experiencing, and would be what the homoeopath calls the *simillimum*. If *Coffea* were given to the patient, her symptoms would subside, whatever their cause.

Or, take the common fever symptoms: dry, red-flushed face, rage, great heat, dilated pupils: this is how someone might be if he had taken the poison belladonna in a crude form, so when this situation emerges in illness the remedy that has the most similar symptom picture will be *Belladonna*, diluted or potentized in the manner customary with homoeopathic medicines. Like is treated with like, which is the basic principle of homoeopathic medicine.

Since the remedy needs to be capable of producing in a healthy person a similar range of symptoms to those manifested in a sick one, it is clear that the homoeopath will need to know both the patient's symptoms and the symptoms which each potential remedy substance can produce in a healthy person, in order to match the person to the remedy. But the homoeopath needs to know more than just the main or presenting complaint or symptom. She needs to know the particular ways in which this complaint is manifesting in this particular person – the special, or peculiar, ways in which the complaint shows itself in each individual.

For instance, the homoeopath might be treating someone whose main complaint was depression. There are many remedies whose symptom picture includes depression, so the homoeopath would seek to establish a more complete picture of the person's individual symptoms before choosing a remedy. If, for example, the person were mentally agitated and inclined to suffer from rheumatic complaints as well as being depressed, then the remedy might well be *Aurum*; if, on the other hand, the person were exhausted and subject to varicose veins and backache during menstruation, as well as being depressed, then the remedy might well be *Sepia*. In some cases the *cause* of the condition is an important indicator: if the person had been depressed after being bereaved and was now unable to move on from the grief, then the remedy might be *Ignatia* or *Natrum muriaticum*.

Any substance at all can be used as a homoeopathic remedy: as long as you know what symptoms it can produce in a healthy person then you know what range of symptoms it can cure in a sick person. Giving a sick person such a remedy supports his vitality (or immune system) and enables him to throw off whatever named disease is current by strengthening his entire defence system, making his body's own system work better.

So the next thing is to decide what the sick person's symptoms are, and to match them to a remedy picture. In order to do this we ask questions and make observations of the person who is ill, formulate a symptom picture and match it to the remedy picture found in the *Materia Medica*, a compendium of symptoms.

Chapter Three

———

THE MEDICINES OF
THE MATERIA MEDICA

The detailed symptom pictures for each homoeopathic medicine are to be found in reference works called **Materia Medica**. These contain records of the effects of remedies on people, derived either from accounts of accidental poisonings, from the 'provings' (reports of experiments using volunteers who have taken the medicines under controlled conditions in order to discover their healing effects), or from clinical reports of the results of treating sick people.

In the early 1800s Samuel Hahnemann began to collect information relating to about 20 remedies, and the process has continued without interruption since then. Nowadays some 3,000 substances have been developed for use as homoeopathic medicines, and detailed information about their action has been and continues to be collected, analysed and constantly up-dated in the light of new clinical evidence.

Anything at all can be used as a homoeopathic remedy as long as it is known what range of symptoms it can cause (and therefore cure). In the early days of homoeopathy most of the remedies were made from plants used in the botanical medicine current in the eighteenth century, such as belladonna, chamomile and aconite, but gradually other substances were brought into use as their potential for healing was recognized.

Sepia, the brown inky liquid disguise put out by fish of the squid family, was tried as a remedy after Hahnemann noticed that a severely depressed painter friend had the habit of sucking his sepia-covered brushes. Through speculating as to whether his friend's depression had been caused by this practice, Hahnemann discovered what was to become one of the most important homoeopathic remedies for people suffering from a whole range of symptoms associated with depression, including apathy, frustration, irritability and exhaustion.

Likewise the poisonous symptoms of *Phosphorus*, a substance used in the making of matches, were beginning to be well known from reports of diseases appearing among match-makers. Its potential as a homoeopathic remedy was soon seen: it can stop haemorrhages, cure various types of blood disorders, and assuage nightmares and depression, among other things.

Over the years the ***Materia Medica*** has been expanded by the addition of remedies made from other plants, trees and minerals, metals such as gold, silver and platinum, disease products such as tuberculous sputum, cancerous tissue, modern chemical drugs such as penicillin and prednizolone, and even substances such as chocolate. These medicines are subjected to 'provings' to ascertain their action before they are used as true homoeopathic remedies.

In provings healthy volunteers, or 'provers', take controlled doses of certain substances until they begin to produce the symptoms of the drug in themselves. They then record both the gross and subtle effects in minute detail. The provers of *Arsenicum*, for example, took the poison in tiny doses over a period of time and discovered that not only did they begin to feel weak and lose their skin colour – features of arsenic poisoning which had been known for centuries – but also that they became 'anxiously impatient', 'vexed about trifles' and could not 'leave off talking of the faults of others'. The subtle psychological effects of the remedy were recorded in just as much detail as the physical symptoms, and it is for this reason that homoeopathy was and is able to use such emotional symptoms in the process of choosing a remedy.

As the use of the medicines in practice has increased over the last hundred years, so the information from the provings has been augmented both by further provings and by information gained from extensive clinical use. What was noted in the provings as a passing symptom, a transitory effect of *Arsenicum*, 'vexed about trifles', can now be seen to be a strong character trait of a person who often needs the remedy *Arsenicum*, a person who is likely to be more than ordinarily meticulous and conscientious as well as quickly vexed.

The remedy pictures found in the various *Materia Medica* start out, then, merely as lists of symptoms derived from provings and poisonings, expanded by symptoms described in clinical practice. The material is presented in different ways in different versions of the *Materia Medica*, each presentation an attempt to give some form to the overpowering mass of detail provided by the original listing of symptoms. Each picture is designed to increase understanding, and varies in its emphasis and detail according to the particular focus of the writer.

The *Materia Medica* in this book includes pictures of 21 substances, some of the remedies most widely used and readily available in homoeopathy today. In my short descriptions I have concentrated on giving a general 'psychological profile' of each remedy, a profile which includes most of the symptoms characteristic of or special to the emotional disposition represented in each remedy picture.

As interest in the psychological and emotional make-up of human beings has increased, so more attention has been paid to these aspects in homoeopathic medicine, and we are now developing more detailed pictures of the psychological and emotional symptoms of many remedies which I have been able to draw on in this book.

I have also included in the descriptions many of the characteristic physical symptoms, as these are essential guides to the remedy. They will help you confirm which remedy is needed, because even when you are looking primarily at psychological or emotional conditions you need to match the important physical symptoms of remedy and person, to maintain the essential aspect of directing the cure to the *whole person*.

It will be obvious that since I have selected 21 out of a corpus of 3,000 remedies, I have had to leave out a lot of very important remedies. This book cannot cover the whole range of homoeopathic medicine; it is just a 'taster'.

Remedy Pictures

If you try to absorb all the details of a remedy picture at once you will sink without trace under a mass of apparently unrelated details. The provings of some of the major remedies have brought out thousands of symptoms in all areas of the body. Reading a complete picture of a remedy is like looking at one of Pieter Brueghel's paintings: there is far too much going on to be able to take everything in. Every time you go back to the picture you will find something else in it. However, the fact is that if you have any knowledge at all of what the painting looks like, you will never mistake a painting by Brueghel for one by Monet. You know straightaway that Monet would not have painted a dark people-covered icy lake, and that Brueghel would not have painted a sunlit lily-covered one. Even without being art critics we unconsciously absorb what is characteristic of the style of each painter. Likewise we will always be able to tell a crow from a robin, even if we know very little about birds. We see what is characteristic about each bird: in this case each one's colour and size. It is the same with remedies.

If you look, for instance, at the picture of *Pulsatilla* in the *Materia Medica*, you will find that a person needing this remedy when ill is likely to be a fairly people-dependent kind of person, enjoying company and sometimes becoming needy, weepy and clingy. He is also likely to feel physically chilly, but at the same time to be uncomfortable in a stuffy room and quite badly affected by heat. He may faint easily and probably will rarely feel thirst at all.

If you look at the picture of *Arsenicum* you will see that a person needing this remedy will appear predominantly anxious and busy; she is also likely to feel better if she has company, but will not cry so easily; she may be meticulously tidy and precise in thoughts and dress. She too will be a chilly person but will feel better for being in a warm room or exposed to direct heat. She will be thirsty, not for huge cups of tea, but will drink little and often through the day.

A person needing *Natrum muriaticum* will generally be a quiet, reserved sort of person, will probably not want company at all, will definitely not want sympathy or comfort from others and will certainly not let them see him cry. He will not have a marked temperature preference but will be generally quite thirsty. You might notice that his bottom lip is cracked in the middle.

These sketches attempt to communicate the symptoms which are characteristic of each remedy, most of which should be present in order for that remedy to be useful.

Just as a picture of a dramatic single tree probably would not have been painted by Brueghel, and just as a small bird with a red breast could not be a crow, a person in a *Pulsatilla* state is quite unlikely to be comfortable in a warm room, and someone in an *Arsenicum* state cannot really be happy alone when ill.

HOMOEOPATHIC SYMPTOMS

Remedy pictures include a wide range of what homoeopaths call symptoms, a word used with a wider meaning in homoeopathy than in orthodox medicine. While some of these are clearly unhealthy – 'impulse to kill', 'loathing of life', 'waking at night thinking she will die' – others may seem to be scarcely more than character traits: 'bad-tempered in the mornings', 'reserved', 'easily moved to tears'. Remedy pictures traditionally include a blend of symptoms covering a range of intensity of illness, and obviously people may express symptoms anywhere on a spectrum ranging from seeming personality traits to severe mental breakdown. Different types of symptoms may be important at different stages of prescribing.

Because of this it is useful to distinguish in homoeopathic medicine between two approaches to prescribing, commonly referred to as *constitutional* and *acute*.

Many homoeopaths form what is known as a constitutional picture of both patients and remedies. These pictures reflect a person's basic way of being both in health and disease, a way which is more or less in balance in health and gets progressively more exaggerated and unbalanced in disease. So someone having a *Pulsatilla* constitution would be likely to enjoy company generally, be of a mild and pleasant disposition, be easily emotional, chilly and thirstless when he is in reasonable health. When ill (acute stage), however, he might develop catarrhal symptoms more readily than other types might, would tend to feel sick after eating fatty foods, would have bad circulation with white fingertips or chilblains, and would tend to have trouble with his veins. Emotionally he might break down in spells of uncontrollable weeping and become rather over-dependent (even demanding) on company and support. At a later stage he might fear a complete breakdown, be terrified to leave the safety of the house and have panic attacks when left alone. At an even later stage he might develop fear of insanity and suffer obsessional religious ideas and delusions of persecution. All these symptoms would belong to the *Pulsatilla* picture but represent different degrees of ill-health within it. We might use the expression '*Pulsatilla* type' to refer to a person manifesting this constellation of characteristics and symptoms.

A *Phosphorus* type, when healthy, might be very sociable and entertaining, the life and soul of any party, might crave fish and chocolate and be a little on the chilly side, and might perhaps be inclined to get nose-bleeds. When ill she would be likely to develop bronchitis or bad coughs, suffer from internal bleeding and become 'high' or depressed, and also have trouble keeping normal social boundaries between herself and other people, spilling over everywhere emotionally. At a later stage she might develop diabetes or multiple sclerosis, be hypo-manic or feel so exhausted and burnt out that she would be terribly depressed and empty. At an even later stage she might go over into manic-depressive psychosis.

A person's general way of being might correspond to a remedy picture even when she is healthy (and to its more serious manifestations when she is ill), or she might fit a particular remedy picture only when she is suffering from an acute illness. That is to say, a person may be generally constitutionally sensitive to and susceptible of being helped by a particular remedy, or only temporarily sensitive to it during an acute illness. In the first instance the person's *type* may be said to correspond to the remedy picture; in the second the person's *state* may be said to correspond to the remedy picture. In either case, the person will benefit whenever the way in which her body/mind is reacting to 'dis-ease' resembles the picture of the remedy.

For instance, people of many different basic constitutions or make-ups or types may well need *Ignatia* when bereaved, because the *Ignatia* symptom picture is preeminently that of the confused and emotional state which touches most people for a while in the first stages of grief: alternately weeping openly and shutting oneself off, laughing inappropriately, often at serious things, sighing, sometimes sleepless, sometimes over-sleeping, lashing out in sudden short bursts of anger, wishing things were different from the way they are.

There are also people who may be said to have a basically *Ignatia* character or constitution. This type of person is usually described as being an idealist, someone who always wants perfection, has difficulty in reconciling herself to the ordinary or the less than ideal, always wishing things were different and greatly susceptible to the influence of loss in her life, whether through death or through disappointment in love.

A homoeopathic remedy probably acts most deeply when it matches both the acute illness and the person's basic constitution. However, it can do wonders when correctly prescribed for the acute state only, and can often clear the picture so well that the person's true constitutional state comes into focus.

It is sometimes assumed that a person will display only one constitutional remedy picture throughout life. However, this is rarely the case. Most people conform to the pictures of a number of closely related remedies at various times during their lives. We are all multiple personalities in some ways.

The image you see of any given person at any given time conforms to what is sometimes called the *persona*, the dominant way a person presents himself to the world, how he thinks of himself. Then, of course, the more you get to know a person the more aspects of him you begin to see and the fuller your picture of him becomes. The art of homoeopathic prescribing is to prescribe for the clearest picture you have of a person, and then to wait and see what happens.

Chapter Four

SELECTING THE REMEDY

The successful prescribing of homoeopathic remedies is based on matching the picture of the remedy that will cure to the picture of the person who is ill. The picture does not have to match exactly, it just has to be similar; the more similar, the better the chance it has of exerting its catalytic effect on the patient's self-healing system. So the homoeopath's first task is to establish a picture of the important symptoms of the sick person.

All symptoms are potentially important and it might seem, when a homoeopath takes your history before prescribing for you, that she wants to know everything about you. This is not the case, but she will want to know everything that is characteristic of you, everything that represents your individual way of manifesting whatever disease is present at the moment, and this includes being interested in the way you describe your symptoms, the way you talk, your general attitude to life, and a lot of your characteristics (which may seem to you to have nothing to do with your illness).

As will be clear from what has been discussed already, a homoeopathic symptom picture encompasses more aspects of a person than those which orthodox medicine associates with disease. It attempts to depict everything of significance that is taking place within the person who is ill at the time of the illness. Whatever is happening is an expression of just one state of dis-ease, one illness. All the symptoms present are related to each other, expressing a single mind–body condition. Everything about the person is, or may be, a clue to the remedy.

Suppose that your child is having terrible tantrums. She just won't calm down. This might be an indication in homoeopathic terms for *Aconite*, *Calcarea carbonica*, *Stramonium*, *Belladonna*, *Chamomilla* or *Ignatia*, to name but a few. How do you decide which to give her?

Look at what else is going on as well as the tantrums: What seems to have caused them? What is her body temperature like? What has she just eaten? What other symptoms has she got? Always look at the bigger picture, as complete a picture as possible. If the tantrum takes the form of not wanting something she asked for only a moment ago, and is accompanied by unbelievable rage, then think of *Chamomilla*. If she is banging her head on the walls and seems affected by bright light, then think of *Stramonium*. If the tantrum is caused by fever and is accompanied by overheating, then think of *Belladonna*.

This is one of the hardest things to grasp initially about homoeopathy, that sometimes symptoms which appear to have nothing to do with the most obvious problem are more useful when choosing the right remedy. However, once you grasp this principle it makes everything simple. Treat the person, not the disease. Is the person ill in a *Belladonna* way or a *Pulsatilla* way?

What helps us to choose the right remedy is the peculiar – that is, special, personal and distinctive – way in which the patient reacts to the illness, in the whole of his person and personality: feelings, behaviour, body temperature, appetite, etc., for example.

The most important thing to look for is probably the way the person is at the moment. What is his personality here and now? How does this person seem to you in this moment? Is he afraid, depressed, cheerful? Timid, stolid, competitive? Open, reserved? Does he talk quickly or slowly? Is he confident or shy?

The principle is always the same: try to match as much as possible of the person's picture in illness to a remedy picture. You should put more emphasis on his general state than on his particular complaints, that is, put more emphasis on his emotional disposition, general mood, body temperature, appetite, thirst, on the general way he behaves than on the particular named illness from which he appears to be suffering.

What you are looking for is the marked characteristic features of the patient when ill, which, of course, encompass some of his constant characteristic features when either well or ill. You then match these to the marked characteristic features of the remedies which you will find in the *Materia Medica*. Using this approach you will discover that some people often need the same remedy whenever they are ill, whatever the precise nature of the named disease, because of their individual and characteristic way of responding to illness, no matter what it is.

When thinking about a person to whom you plan to give a remedy it is important to try to perceive her normal way of being and then to try to assess how she has changed since she has been ill. So, for example, you might see a person whom you know well, who is normally an organized, efficient pleasant individual, a hard worker, a bit of a worrier, someone, nevertheless, who gets on with things. Another time you might find this person depressed and anxious, fed up and overworked, worrying pointlessly about her health. Both these pictures would correspond to the remedy picture of *Arsenicum*, but to *Arsenicum* at different stages of disruption of health: the first at quite a minor stage, the second at a more serious stage, though not as severe as if the friend were displaying quite paranoid symptoms, imagining that you hated her and were trying to kill her by putting something in her food, all major *Arsenicum* symptoms but belonging to a state of more advanced disruption of health.

Every homoeopathic remedy works on both the psychological and physical level at once. The most efficient way to select the remedy, even when the disruption in health with which you are directly concerned seems to be emotional rather than physical, is to try to reflect both the emotional and important physical symptoms in your choice of remedy, try to mirror back the broadest picture of the disorganization in the vital force or energy field of the patient. Homoeopathic treatment is a process of restoring harmony to the person's nature, not of simply removing one or two symptoms that are inconvenient or painful.

Although all symptoms are useful and contribute to the formation of the complete picture, there are two particularly important types of symptom to look for when selecting a remedy: what homoeopaths call *general* symptoms and what they call *characteristic* symptoms.

General Symptoms

General symptoms are those which affect the whole person, as opposed to particular symptoms which affect only a part. So, for instance, it is a general symptom to feel the cold, a particular one to have cold feet, a general symptom to suffer from burning pains anywhere in the body, a particular symptom to have a burning pain in the throat or the big toe. We are used to concentrating on particular symptoms in orthodox medicine, but in homoeopathy we concentrate on the symptoms that give us the best sense of how the person as a whole reacts to dis-ease, not just how one diseased part of the person is reacting at the present time.

Characteristic Symptoms

Characteristic symptoms are those which tend to individualize a remedy picture – for instance, *Ignatia*'s general tendency to express contradictory symptoms: to feel better for eating indigestible things, to feel hot in cold weather; or *Pulsatilla*'s general changeability: when you find yourself saying: 'I don't know what remedy's needed here because the symptoms keep changing,' think of *Pulsatilla*. These symptoms are like the red of a robin's breast, they signal *Ignatia* or *Pulsatilla* quite immediately. Because of their importance they are sometimes known as 'keynotes' of the remedy, notes around which the tune of the remedy is constructed.

All the remedies are variations on different ways of expressing emotions and attitudes common to all human beings. So all the remedy pictures represent most human emotions in different proportions and with different emphases. For instance, *Arsenicum* manifests more anxiety than *Phosphorus*, *Phosphorus* more spontaneity and less stamina than *Arsenicum*; *Natrum muriaticum* is more reserved than most, *Nux vomica* more irritable. Some remedy pictures tend to get oversimplified so that, for instance, *Sulphur* is said to be 'lazy and selfish', *Arsenicum* 'anxious and critical', *Pulsatilla* 'mild and tearful'. Often you can use these simple descriptions as a rough guide to the remedy, but just as often you need to observe more closely and get a true sense of the personality of both the remedy *and* of the person to whom you are trying to fit this remedy.

Remedy pictures depict personality characteristics across a spectrum, from normal healthy behaviour with a characteristic emphasis (like the fastidiousness of *Arsenicum* or the enthusiasm of *Phosphorus*), through to the more rigid representations of these fundamental attitudes which are present in illness (persistent orderliness or constant instability of mood, for instance), to even more distorted versions which appear in states of near or actual breakdown: obsession or mania.

The art of distinguishing between remedy pictures is to learn to see how each remedy represents basic personality differences at different stages of illness. In the pages that follow some 21 remedies are dealt with in detail, and attention paid to ways of distinguishing between them in their differing modes of expressing illness *and* in the different stages of illness.

Chapter Five

———

CHOOSING THE POTENCY

At this point we need to look briefly at the question of what exactly a remedy is. So far we have been referring to it as if it were precisely the same as the substance from which it is derived. However, by the time we prescribe a remedy in homoeopathic medicine we are no longer using merely a herbal or a chemical substance, the plant aconite or the element sulphur for instance, but we are also including in our prescription the energetic field around those substances: we are prescribing not aconite itself but the energy of aconite, if you like. This energy is made accessible by the process of preparation invented by Hahnemann.

Although in the early days of his practice Hahnemann prescribed crude doses of medicines, as did all doctors, he soon became aware of the importance of prescribing much smaller doses in consideration of the fact that he was prescribing on the *similia* principle – the principle that 'like cures like' – and because he was providing remedies that could *cause* what he was proposing to cure. It became important not to give too much of a medicine so as not to risk exacerbating the condition he was trying to make better. Early on, therefore, Hahnemann began to dilute his medicines, and gradually realized that the weaker doses not only had a less damaging impact on the patient, but were also actually much more effective in bringing about a cure. Encouraged by this observation, he continued to experiment and discovered that the medicines became even more powerful if they were not only diluted but shaken up vigorously ('succussed') during the process of dilution.

He himself thought that the remedies increased in power as a result of this process because he had managed to release some of the energy of the substance, some of its 'spirit' or 'vital force', as he put it. The process and its effects are still far from being fully understood, but it is important to bear in mind that the action of a homoeopathic remedy is dynamic in some way rather than merely chemical or herbal, and that the remedies are more powerful, more energetic, deeper acting, the more they have been diluted and succussed in this way, the more they have been 'potentized'.

The least-potentized remedies are the ones generally available in pharmacists and health food stores: these are conventionally sold in the 6th or the 30th potency. The fact that the potency is lower does not mean that the remedy will be less powerful – when they match the symptoms low-potency remedies can be very powerful – but it does mean that the effects may be shorter-lived and that you may have to take the tablet quite frequently to maintain its positive effect. Much higher potencies, ranging from 30 to well over 100,000 are available from specialist pharmacies and can be prescribed by professional homoeopaths, though, in fact, many professional homoeopaths never use them. It is best to stay within the low band of potencies (6–30) until you gain some experience of using them. (If you have any difficulty obtaining remedies locally you can order them directly from the specialist pharmacies listed in Appendix Two.)

With most remedies and for most conditions it is probably a good idea to start prescribing with the 6th potency and eventually to move up to the 12th and then the 30th when you are more confident. The lower the potency the more likely the remedy is to need frequent repetition, so if you are prescribing mostly in 6s, 12s or 30s you may have to repeat the process more often than some homoeopaths, who may give you a single remedy in the 10,000th potency (10m) and tell you to come back in a couple of months.

When you have decided what remedy you are going to give and in what potency, give just one dose, or one tablet. Try not to touch the tablet: either tip it from the cap of the bottle into the person's mouth or tip it into her mouth from a clean piece of paper or spoon. The person receiving the remedy should then suck the tablet for a few minutes or chew it if it is very hard. Do not eat, drink, brush your teeth or smoke 15–20 minutes before and after taking a tablet. If you should accidentally drop any tablets, throw them away. All these precautions are taken simply to protect the remedy from being made useless by being contaminated with strong smells, tastes or dirt. If you make a mistake it will not be in anyway dangerous.

If you want homoeopathic remedies to work at their best and if you want to be clear that they have indeed worked, you should try not to take other medicines at the same time. However, it is not always possible to be purist about this and you should *never* stop taking a prescribed orthodox medicine without first consulting your doctor or a health practitioner. It is quite safe to take homoeopathic remedies at the same time as other medicines and the remedies usually work to some extent in these circumstances, but they obviously have to work harder and their action may be obstructed by that of the orthodox medicine.

Give the Remedy and Wait

When you have given the remedy, be prepared to wait a while and watch for any reaction. Homoeopathic remedies can work extraordinarily quickly, or they can take time to act. The hardest thing is to be patient in prescribing. However, do not be over-cautious about waiting for the remedy to act if the situation is urgent.

Urgent/Acute

If you are prescribing for an acute condition then you should expect results quite soon if you have chosen the right remedy. There should be some quickly observable lessening of the strength of the symptom in, for instance, a panic attack, a child's angry tantrum, an adult's anticipatory anxiety. I have known someone to start singing around the house within minutes of taking a remedy for anxiety, and a child's tantrum to dissolve like magic.

When the organism is in crisis it takes up the appropriate remedy very quickly. If, in such a case, you have given the chosen remedy three times within half an hour without a clear effect, then reconsider the remedy and, if it still seems right, use a higher potency. If you think you need a higher potency than the one you have, dissolve a tablet in a glass of water (preferably sterilized or mineral water, but use anything in an emergency) and take sips from that, stirring vigorously between each sip. Each sip should be regarded as a dose, and no new dose should be taken till the effect of the last has worn off.

A homoeopathic remedy sometimes works directly and quickly on the symptoms, in which case there will be no doubt about whether it has been effective. At other times, however, the first effect noticed will be an increase in vitality or sense of well-being rather than a direct relief of particular symptoms. This is an excellent sign; it means that the remedy is working. Don't repeat the remedy as long as this sense of feeling good remains. Take more only when you need it – that is, as soon as the symptoms which had improved return, or as soon as the sense of well-being leaves you.

Long-Standing

If, on the other hand, the condition or state you are treating is long-standing, you should not necessarily expect to see results until you have taken the remedy, say, twice a day for a week in the 6th potency.

It is very difficult to give instructions about how to manage homoeopathic potencies: it is mainly a matter of observation and common sense. In general, remember that you are merely trying to get the body's self-healing system to act on its own behalf, not to take over for it.

So give the remedy just as much as you need to start this process. Once the process has started do not repeat the remedy until its action has ceased and the patient's improvement stalls or stops. In a long-standing complaint you may have to repeat the remedy frequently to maintain the improvement.

Very often in complaints or conditions that are defined as being primarily emotional you will find that professional homoeopaths will use high-potency remedies whose effects tend to be longer-lasting than those of the lower potencies. However, this does not mean that highly effective treatment cannot take place with low-dose remedies given more frequently.

It is not dangerous to take too many homoeopathic remedies,

merely pointless as they work better the more gently and sparingly they are used. If a remedy does not work (because the correct one has not been chosen), nothing will happen, nothing will improve. Occasionally, if you take too much either in terms of potency or the number of tablets, you may experience an aggravation or slight worsening of symptoms. This will be short-lived and can be made even shorter by drinking strong coffee to negate the remedy's action. Such an aggravation is nothing to worry about, however, and is even a good sign in that it usually precedes an improvement in symptoms.

A very few people are particularly sensitive to the action of the remedies and may overreact to many of them. Nevertheless they will usually be able to find a way (perhaps with the help of a professional homoeopath) of taking remedies so that such an overreaction does not take place.

Chapter Six

_____

PSYCHOLOGICAL
AND EMOTIONAL PROBLEMS

Finally, before coming to consider specific problems, let us look at the central issue of this book, the question of psychological and emotional health. How do psychological and emotional dispositions arise? How do the emotional differences between people arise? We all observe the subtle differences in children from the moment of birth, even children of the same parents, even identical twins will have some differences of temperament and personality from each other, and these differences will develop more and more as time goes on.

Some of the differences are clearly genetic, others will arise as individuals are affected by slightly different circumstances in life and as they react or adapt to these circumstances. The different ways in which we react to life events, the varying adaptive modes we adopt may, gradually, as we use them over and over again, become crystallized into a sort of protective shield.

These protective shields correspond to what are called 'complexes' or 'defence systems' or 'subpersonalities' by various systems of psychotherapy. In homoeopathy they correspond to some of the emotional aspects of a remedy picture. In other words, a remedy picture in its emotional aspects is a representation of one or more psychological survival systems. We may all have several such systems within us and find that we use one or more of them more frequently than others, developing a core of subpersonalities which we come to regard as ourselves but which are really only aspects of ourselves.

For example, the *Arsenicum* subpersonality or survival system is the part of us which needs to keep everything in order, be meticulously accurate; the *Natrum muriaticum* subpersonality is the part of us that needs to be reserved, closed, keep people out; the *Phosphorus* subpersonality is the part of us which wants to relate, to be the life and soul of the party. We all contain within us these aspects and many more, but we tend to get restricted to playing just one or two or a few more of these roles. Some of them have become really important to us and we cannot imagine being without them, even if they cause us pain.

Usually these little survival systems work well for a while but then they stop working so well. Usually symptoms or illness develop when the subpersonality that is in the foreground, our main survival mode, is no longer appropriate to our current circumstances.

For instance, your childhood may have been such that you developed a very orderly, precise way of functioning, a need to be in control (*Arsenicum*). You may have had to do this because your family home was chaotic. The home you live in now, however, may be much more relaxed and you could, if you dared, trust your current family, but the habit of mistrust and self-protection is blocking you off from really relaxing. Having a strongly developed *Arsenicum* pattern is no longer useful to you, yet you still may find it difficult to abandon.

One of the things taking a remedy will do is help you to drop these out-of-date defensive systems. People say that they feel much more relaxed, do not have to fill up every minute with work, find themselves no longer hypercritical of the children. It is not that you lose all your character, can no longer do all the things you used to, but there is no longer the distortion surrounding your actions. You are not so tense about being who you are.

Another way of looking at it is to say that we have all acquired several messages or scripts during our lives, sets of internalized instructions as to who we are and how we should be. For a while these are useful but what happens is that we forget to change the scripts when they become inappropriate.

It can often be difficult to cure or attempt to change an emotional cast of mind. People are very often attached to their emotional symptoms in a way that they are not attached to their physical ones.

We identify our emotional symptoms as 'us' far more than we do physical symptoms, and this can make attempting a cure very difficult. There is often a fear that if some psychological imbalance is balanced out or smoothed we'll lose some of our personality. If we're not manic we won't be good company (we think), if we're not obsessionally tidy we won't be good housewives, if we don't work compulsively for 18 hours a day we won't be responsible.

As long as they are still needed, still appropriate, then these protective subpersonalities may not be curable with homoeopathy. In these cases, as with other resistant cases in homoeopathy, we have first to remove the 'maintaining cause', to pinpoint why the protective mode is still appropriate – a poor current relationship, perhaps, or an overdemanding boss? Often at this point we need to bring in the help of psychotherapy or counselling. This may help remove the fear of change by giving us insight into the origins and development of our original subpersonalities.

A homoeopathic remedy picture is, then, in some respects, a depiction of a survival system, represented in the energy of a particular substance. We use the remedy to mirror the particular survival mode in which a person's life is represented, for the moment.

For a long time psychological and emotional problems have been difficult to talk about. There is some sort of stigma attached to being depressed or anxious that is not attached to having a heart condition or asthma. People who suffer with their nerves try to pretend to their friends that they don't. However, there seems to be a change taking place in this area and it is becoming slightly more socially acceptable to admit to being emotionally upset or ill.

In many ways this is a good thing: it means people can be honest about what is happening to them and may even be able to take time off work because they are grieving or exhausted or depressed, rather than having to pretend they have flu. This is already happening in some jobs.

In other ways, however, this has led to the medicalization of emotions and the increased involvement of the medical profession as experts in the field of ordinary human feelings. In many cases the breakdown of social and community networks of support also has led to our putting the means for solving problems such as loneliness or misery into the hands of experts instead of being able to find enough peer support to be able to sort out/come to terms with our problems ourselves, without drugs. This is unfortunate, but it is not a moral defect for anyone to need help.

One very important thing that learning to use homoeopathy can do is help us to take back our own power to help ourselves, to influence our own states of emotions without having to submit to the sometimes personality-destroying power of the medical system and the drug companies.

PART TWO

Help Is at Hand

Chapter Seven

DEPRESSION
AND SUICIDAL THOUGHTS

It is, unfortunately, a common human experience to feel low-spirited, despondent, gloomy, hopeless, melancholy: it is because of this that the feelings associated with depression are the subject of a great deal of moving literature, art and music. They may emerge in response to life events that are difficult to bear: the death of a lover, friend or relative, the break-up of an important relationship, the experience of being trapped in an unfulfilling job, or of being made redundant, or being in the throes of some spiritual or moral crisis. Or they may seem to come from nowhere, out of the blue, for no apparent reason.

Although there are very few people who do not get depressed at some time in their lives, the experience is no less painful for being common. It is probably the most difficult of all human emotions to bear because the sufferer usually feels so completely alone in it, completely cut off from other people, however willing they are to help. When we are depressed we seem to watch others as if we were standing alone in the cold outside a lighted house, unable to go in. Or else we feel as if trapped inside our own dark and empty house, unable to make a move to those outside.

When we are depressed we feel untouchable, sometimes even dangerous; parents characteristically feel that their children would be better off without them, would be safer; I have known someone who felt like a piece of nuclear waste, capable of contaminating the whole world. When depressed we feel useless and worthless, guilty of some unknown but terrible crime; there seems no way to resolve the situation and no point. It feels as if it will last forever and that the only way to end it is by death. We talk about feeling empty inside, as if there were a hole inside us, as if we were on the edge of a deep pit, enveloped in a mass of grey cloud. We can feel it around us and inside us, we can almost touch it as it settles over us. Life feels completely meaningless, pointless. It's all hopeless.

We can pretend, of course. We pretend a lot of the time. We have to protect our families, our jobs. The ability to put on a front sometimes makes us feel that we're even pretending to be depressed, but we're not. As soon as the need to pretend has gone then there we are, balancing on the edge of the pit again. Eventually we may not be able to pretend anymore and we may just sit and stare or stay in bed or attempt suicide or get drunk or go missing. Recovering is difficult because it doesn't feel safe to be happy. What if it comes back? It won't last. When we are happy the fear of a relapse is always lurking. We have to be careful all the time in case it comes back. The slightest lick of the cloud round our edges and we are terrified.

Deep depression like this is a terrible state to be in and the sufferer will need a lot of help and support to move out of it. Often this is just what a depressed person does not get because friends find it distressing and frightening to be around someone who is depressed and cannot accept help, and eventually, after being rebuffed several times, either try to ignore it, hope it will pass, try and get the sufferer to shake it off in some way, or get him to go to the doctor and get some pills: anything to try to make this alien and alienating state go away.

There are many theories about the causes of depression, but no single clear explanation has emerged. Sometimes it seems to have its origin in unresolved problems from childhood, like many of our emotional difficulties. Sometimes there seems to be some chemical cause: hormone imbalance, for example, or interruption to the brain's supply of various necessary chemicals. Sometimes the immediate cause seems clear when, for instance, it comes on as a reaction to something: bereavement, loss of a job, loss of a relationship, diagnosis of serious illness, disappointment in some project. In such cases, when the cause is apparent, other people can sympathize to some extent, though even then a remarkably short space of time is often allowed for recovery from these very traumatic events.

Sometimes it comes on when some long unsorted issue is reactivated. We may not even notice how it happened, but some current event pushes us back many years into what is usually a childhood position of powerlessness. We go back to being three years old, being told off for something we did or did not do, or to a time when something happened that we still feel guilty about. We take an exam and find that we are again in a position of not being able to do it. We get into a situation that unconsciously reminds us of an old pain. These triggers can be difficult to notice and are probably the explanation behind so-called 'out of the blue', 'no reason' depressions.

Sometimes depression may arise because we don't express some other emotion: often anger. We suppress it without realizing it and we get depressed. In some people this is such a habitual pattern they don't even know that they suppress anger, they don't even feel it. Or we suppress hurt: 'That's fine' we say and begin to feel depressed and worthless, almost without noticing.

Sometimes what we call depression is really a state of existential despair, a state of acknowledgment of our own loneliness in the world that we all have to face at some time. Most of us would rather not face it at all, and when these feelings of meaningless become too strong, we rush for the bottle of alcohol or tablets, for a relationship or even a good meal. We'll do anything to avoid the acknowledgment of our essential aloneness.

In the early days of history, depression was seen as due to a loss of power, a theft of the soul by spirits. In early Christian theology, despair was seen as a sin because it was 'wrong' to be unhappy in God's creation; later it was seen as an almost constitutional state, melancholia, a part of the make-up of any human being which was stronger in some than in others. It is only in today's secular world that it has become so clearly categorized as a medical condition. Patients come and say that the doctor has told them they've 'got depression' as if it were something they had caught and which could be treated with an antibiotic.

It seems to be more and more the trend today in orthodox medicine to regard depression as a physical illness, caused by an imbalance or deficiency of certain chemicals in the blood. There is, however, no hard evidence for this: all the research pointing to this simple conclusion is flawed or incomplete. It is odd that this opinion should be coming to the fore at the same time that, for many other forms of illness formerly regarded as entirely physically based, the existence of a strong emotional or psychological component is now generally accepted – in cancer, for instance, or rheumatoid arthritis or ME.

The consequence (or perhaps the cause) of the definition of depression as a physically-based illness has been the emergence of a vast array of drugs to treat it. In the early days of the medical treatment of depression such terrifying treatments as lobotomy (surgical removal of the frontal lobe of the brain) or ECT (electro-convulsive therapy, by which severe shocks were passed through the brain) were used. They both had the same intention: to destroy the parts of the brain which felt conflicting emotions. The earliest modern drugs, the tricyclic anti-depressants, tried to achieve the same effect by chemical means. More recent anti-depressants (such as Nardil) have sought to increase the amount of norepinephrine in the central nervous system, and the latest ones, such as Prozac and Xanax, seek to increase the supply of serotonin to the brain.

From the early tricyclic anti-depressants, through those popular in the sixties, to the serotogenic modern drugs, the story seems to be the same: big claims are made for them, many thousands of people have them prescribed, many people feel no benefit from them, many people feel a little less depressed, a little less suicidal, some people feel a great deal better, many unpleasant side-effects are reported and court cases are pending against the manufacturers of many of these drugs in connection with gross 'side-effects' caused to those taking them.

Although all this is well known, people continue to take anti-depressants. ECT is even making a comeback in some areas. To some degree this is because, when depressed, people are rarely in a position to argue with the medical establishment. They feel powerless and, frankly, so terrible that they are prepared to try anything, even something which might give them only temporary relief. When we feel depressed we often feel very slowed down, sluggish, as if our brain isn't working properly, our sleep is disturbed, and all this makes us susceptible to theories about chemical imbalance, hopeful that perhaps there really is a simple chemical explanation which would relieve us of this terrible state of despair.

The doctors themselves are presumably acting in what they consider to be their patients' best interests, hoping that the drugs will offer some temporary relief, get their patients over a difficult period which might otherwise result in suicide. Depression is a self-limiting condition: if you survive it, you get over it. No one has the time or money to go fully into the problems of a depressed person. Even if the depressed person doesn't want to take the drugs, often the opportunity to take time off work is dependent on getting a certificate from a doctor, who will eventually offer drug treatment and, naturally enough, may be a little restive if his or her patients refuse to take it and continue to get worse.

Another consideration is that, though these drugs may not always make us significantly less depressed, they do seem to work to stop us being quite so anxious: they flatten moods so that the depression is not so severe or disabling. Although they don't deal with the cause they sometimes give the mind a rest and then, by the time we stop taking them, we have got over the depression anyway, until the next time. There is also a certain comfort to be derived from looking at these moods as physically based: it takes away the moral stigma, the requirement to 'pull ourselves together'. In today's age often the medical diagnosis is temporarily beneficial in that it at least gives people permission to stay in the depression for a while: they are described as suffering from an illness and they can be allowed at least as much sympathy and as long a convalescence as is required for a broken leg.

That is what depression is often about: a means of stalling, shutting everything down until you can cope well enough to go on. It should be read like this. It is well known that if you get depressed because of loss and grief and you go back to work too soon the depression will not resolve itself properly, it will remain around. So, if you get depressed for 'no reason at all', look at whether perhaps you are suppressing any grief or any other strong emotion (especially anger) that has come up for any reason.

Sometimes depression is a clue to the fact that you are doing something in your life you should not be doing, either because it doesn't interest you, or, at a deeper level, because it does not really meet all your needs. Or it tells you the same things about a relationship. We are depressed when we have gone down what we recognize to be a blind alley but are trying to avoid turning back because that would cause pain. What are you putting up with in your life that needs to change? Possibly you can't change it, but perhaps you haven't even thought about whether you could or not. Depression is about loss of power. If you can spot where you are losing power you might be able to turn it round.

Observation and common sense, not to speak of subjective experience, show how most forms of depression arise. They arise in reaction to grief and loss; when trapped in a situation which takes away all power or creativity: such as a marriage that is not working, a job that is unfulfilling – any situation where we cannot express anger or frustration. They also arise at landmark birthdays, when people get in touch with the fact that they are ageing, when we are very tired or very ill or faced with terminal illness or when we are subject to psychological stress and conflict, where too much is demanded of us without adequate support. Often being put in such a situation in the present is sufficient cause for depression, sometimes the particular current circumstances will reach back into some similar situation in childhood.

There are, of course, sometimes primarily physical origins for some depressions. Sometimes they arise because we aren't getting the right food for our particular needs, either not enough vitamins or too much of something that disagrees with us, affects our moods: sugar, for instance can have quite a depressing effect on some people. A variety of environmental influences can precipitate depression in some people: recently a new syndrome has been identified called Seasonal Affective Disorder, used to describe the kind of depression that overwhelms some people when they don't get enough sunlight. This may now be treated by sitting under special lights for several hours a day. We all get depressed when we are very tired, and often don't realize how much sheer exhaustion affects us.

Women frequently suffer from transient depression related to the changes in the balance of hormones: this is particularly noticeable before periods, after childbirth and in the menopause. Men also get depressed as a result of hormonal changes and are very prone to depression once they retire. Women are in general more subject to depression or the diagnosis of depression than men, probably because they are more powerless in society, are not as free as men are to change their situation. It is noticeable that men often get angry where women get depressed.

One of the best ways to overcome depression is to understand its causes and roots within you. Not because this will stop you having the feelings but because it will stop you feeling so powerless and gripped by a shapeless monster. In the matter of depression, knowledge is power: understanding the cause of the pain may not take away the pain but it will take away the powerlessness; it will change depression into unhappiness. A number of books have been written to help people with their depression; some are cited in Appendix 1.

Out of depression frequently emerge suicidal thoughts, attempts at suicide and attempts at self-harm. The expression of suicidal thoughts is one of the most frightening things to deal with if you are not in the helping professions. It is not true that people who threaten suicide do not do it. Nor is it true that there is nothing to be done about it.

In most cases suicidal impulses and thoughts are transient. If you can be with the person at the critical time the mood may change and hope will return. Homoeopathic remedies may help at this time. Often, however, there may be such a settled state of despair as to make any hope you offer seem inadequate.

When you are with anyone in a suicidal state it is most important that you communicate that you have recognized the depth of her despair. Do not try to tell her that she has got it wrong. She hasn't: that is how it feels for her in this moment. If she can be sure that you have really understood how bad it is for her then she may be able to move away from the suicidal thoughts. Sometimes people are thinking about suicide, having suicidal thoughts or feelings but really have no intention of acting on the thoughts. That's how they feel but it's not what they're going to do for a variety of reasons. It can help to be clear about that: it helps both the person having the feelings and the person listening to the feelings to give them free expression without being scared of the consequences.

While there are certain things that depressed and suicidal people have in common, each of us gets depressed in our own individual way. The homoeopathic approach to depression is to regard it as an expression, unique to the individual, of an imbalance of energy, an out-of-tuneness of the vitality of a person. What is needed is to find the remedy or remedies whose symptoms most accurately match or mirror the symptoms of the depressed person, in order to bring the energies of the sick person into alignment with the more harmonious energy of the remedy.

The common symptoms of depression are of less importance in selecting the remedy than the individual and distinct way in which each person manifests that blackness and desolation of mood. All remedy pictures include some kind of description of depression since it is a common human experience as well as an illness. The following remedies are probably the most likely to be considered where depression is the most marked symptom. Check the fuller descriptions in the *Materia Medica* to make sure other aspects of the remedy match the symptom picture as well as possible. Remember also that this is only a very small selection of the remedies that might be helpful in depression: if these do not help then consult someone who knows about the other options.

ANACARDIUM ORIENTALE

The anguished depression in this remedy picture seems to emerge from a sense of losing the battle between the good and evil sides of oneself. The person affected by this kind of depression will be very much aware of this battle, experiencing himself as having an angel on one shoulder and a devil on the other.

This person experiences himself as powerless and incompetent, without any self-confidence. He compensates for this by violence towards both others and himself. He seems to seek his own destruction by provoking others, or tries to hurt or destroy himself by knifing or shooting: he wants to injure himself to stop the internal torment, the conflicting voices in his head.

This remedy picture includes a lot of very strong self-destructive thoughts. In the deeply depressive phase the person suffers deep guilt and torment about the salvation of his soul. In this state he may be wild and restless or can lapse exhausted into a stupefied silence.

ARGENTUM NITRICUM

The agitated and restless apprehensive depression apparent in this remedy picture arises from the affected person's feeling that everything will fail, that she has been forsaken. She feels that she is all by herself, without support, that everything she does is wrong and that she cannot succeed. She feels trapped and frustrated. Exhaustion, particularly mental exhaustion, may cause depression, even nervous breakdown.

She may commit suicide on impulse: she will throw herself off a tall building, for instance, just as she might also injure herself impulsively.

ARSENICUM ALBUM

This remedy might best fit the state often called 'agitated depression', where the sufferer will apparently be more anxious than depressed: anxious about his health, fearful of dying perhaps. Illness is, in fact, something likely to precipitate an *Arsenicum* depression, illness from which the person despairs of recovering and as a result might decide to kill himself.

In depression he is anxious, worried, restless, full of self-reproach and guilt; he tends to go over and over past events and conversations, rehearsing what might have been, convinced that he has offended his friends and that they now hate him. He will be very critical, at first of others and eventually of himself. There will be an obsessional, rigid quality about his depression, an unwillingness to leave it alone, a fretting quality. This state may also be brought on by financial worries, or by some failure in his life.

Thoughts of suicide are common and acting on them is likely, because there is enough energy and competence to translate the impulse into action. He may throw himself under a car, use poison or a knife, or even set himself on fire. The danger time will be what is known as 'the low Arsenicum time' (between midnight and 3 a.m.). He may decide to kill himself because his health is failing and he despairs of getting better, because he has lost control of his life.

AURUM METALLICUM

This is one of the most commonly used remedies for depression. Like someone with an *Arsenicum* remedy picture, someone who needs *Aurum* blames herself for everything, thinking her friends and family no longer care about her and that she deserves this. She is probably more passive in the face of it than someone who needs *Arsenicum*, may sit overcome by melancholy, totally withdrawn and self-blaming, brooding over some imagined sin, some awful act of irresponsibility, feeling completely unworthy. However, she blames circumstance and fate rather than other people. She is impossible to reassure or even temporarily distract, is obsessively preoccupied with self-reproach, and feelings of unworthiness, suicide, death and dying. Classical music usually makes her feel much better.

She may also have periods of more frantic and anxious restless anger mixed with the depression, with angry reproach of herself and rage against circumstance. Suicidal thoughts (and actions) are frequent. It shows the most suicidal disposition in the *Materia Medica*. She worries and plans internally until one day she gives way to the impulse to jump from a height or to run the car off the road; she has obsessive fantasies about committing suicide.

Depression of this type is nearly always the result of sudden or shocking loss: disappointment in love, collapse of a business, bereavement. Abuse of alcohol may also cause depression (or depression may cause abuse of alcohol). It may be worse in the dark or in the Spring.

CALCAREA CARBONICA

The depression of this type is a collapse as much as a depression, and often comes about after a long period of overextending oneself. This person will have struggled to cope and keep things going, to do everything that is needed, to be responsible for everything, and now he simply hasn't the energy, mental or physical, to go on any more. As with an *Aurum* depression, this person will sit staring fixedly, looking heavy and dull, completely unable to make any effort. He broods over what seem like small things, and may repeat mindless actions like counting pins, paper clips or other small objects. He will close himself down completely, yet this state is the fulfilment of his fear that he may be going insane and he will try to hide the fact.

Restlessness and peevishness may be present. He does not have very strong impulses to suicide but these might arise simply from despair and from not wanting to live like this anymore, as with *Arsenicum*. Depression may be worse in the Spring and when it's dark.

IGNATIA AMARA

This depression will show itself in the typical *Ignatia* way: the person will clearly be affected, either quiet and withdrawn but visibly struggling to control her feelings, or obviously and even loudly distressed. Laughter and tears often alternate. The depression is usually an extension of grief and precipitated by loss, either a death or the break-up of a relationship, and usually will not last very long in this intensely agitated form. If it does then think about *Natrum muriaticum*. Music often improves the mood. There is a danger of suicide in this depression because there is energy and passion involved at the height of the acute distress, especially because for a while the sufferer simply cannot imagine living without the person she loves; she thinks her own life worthless if she is abandoned.

LACHESIS

The depressed person, normally lively and active, may become withdrawn and, convinced that he has been betrayed, trusts no one. He fears that people are out to get him. He may also reproach himself severely and fall into aggressive self-criticism. He can descend into complete hopelessness, dullness, apathy and despondency, with a passionate longing for death.

There is usually, however, some energy in a *Lachesis* depression and this can be dangerous because the person may take up some kind of self-destructive activity: cutting himself, drinking heavily, taking drugs, having powerful suicidal impulses.

This depression can be brought on by grief or by failure, by being frustrated in some passionately desired project, or by personal rejection. It can also be associated with the menopause and with any time when there is a loss of sexual libido, with any time when expression is denied; it may also be brought on by abuse of alcohol. It may be much worse in the Spring.

Lachesis is one of the main remedies for people with exaggerated mood swings, where periods of high activity and creativity alternate with periods of flatness and despondency, and for the even more exaggerated manic-depressive states, where depression alternates with elation, despair with mania.

LYCOPODIUM CLAVATUM

The depression characteristic of this remedy will probably be more apparent as the person becomes older: anxiety may be the clearer problem in a younger person. The depression may come on as part of a mid-life crisis, when the person has to confront the fact that all her attempts to succeed beyond her abilities have come to nothing, that she hasn't the energy to keep up her front anymore, that now she will be exposed or found out. She has run out of energy, become despondent, tired of life, wants to be by herself, withdraws into what looks like a haughty self-sufficiency but is really a helpless isolation which, if the person is religious at all, embraces feelings of unworthiness in the sight of her god. It may be worse in the Spring.

NATRUM MURIATICUM

The *Natrum muriaticum* depression may be so well concealed that it is not recognized at all. The person who is depressed tends to mask personal feelings by extending them to the universal, and may simply regard depression as the human condition. He will certainly prefer to be depressed alone, mulling over the past, dwelling on painful memories, nursing hurts, rejecting sympathy or consolation for fear that it is not real. He may suffer from chronic guilt, hoarding his memories of injury and self-condemnation, unwilling to have them taken from him. There may be occasional flashes of gallows humour, black jokes about despair. In certain stages laughing and crying may alternate, in which case it can seem to be an *Ignatia* state of depression.

The depression may be permanent – a sort of pessimistic, melancholy attitude to life in general, a chronic state of tiredness of life, of longing for death: 'I wouldn't commit suicide but I don't mind if I die.'

This particular kind of depression is commonly the result of anger turned inwards and often the long-term consequence of unresolved grief, which may be triggered by childbirth or a death or loss of love. It can come on after shock or grief. It is usually worse in the Spring: while the rest of the world recovers from Winter, *Natrum muriaticum* cannot leave it behind.

NUX VOMICA

The depression in this remedy picture is sometimes obscured by the anger and irritability which characterize it. The person is more likely to blame others than herself, more likely to fight or bluster her way out of a problem than be overwhelmed by despair. However, when these aggressive tactics fail or exhaustion from overwork makes them impossible, severe depression mixed with anger and indignation can follow.

The depression may be brought on by some failure or imagined insult, by some wound to self-respect or by staring inevitable failure in the face. The person usually continues to be irritable and restless, critical and demanding, and there may be spasmodic but violent impulses to suicide. If she can't express her aggression and drive outwardly she may have the impulse to turn it on herself: however, these feelings are rarely acted upon because the person's fear of physical suffering and strong instinct for life prevails over the short-lived impulse characteristic of this remedy picture. The person wants to commit suicide but is afraid to die.

PHOSPHORUS

A deep withdrawn dejection is the opposite side of the coin of the better known *Phosphorus* warmth and outgoingness: *Phosphorus* can sink into a deep loathing of life, the depths of despondency and suicidal despair. The sufferer may become very withdrawn, unwilling to socialize, go out or do anything at all; he may become completely apathetic and indifferent.

This may be the result of exhaustion (burn-out is a classic feature of the *Phosphorus* picture) or from too-rapid growth in adolescence, or it may be a consequence of ageing, when the person becomes convinced that no one will like him now he is losing his looks and energy.

It may be part of a pattern of mood swings in some people, one element in a regular variation between excitement and depression which may verge on the manic-depressive syndrome, as in *Lachesis*, but the mood will not be so passionate and dark and deep, rather lighter and more airy, more suggestive of a butterfly than a snake.

PLATINUM METALLICUM (PLATINA)

People needing *Platina* are often 'moody': they can be sad and weepy one minute and then suddenly laughing and apparently happy in a way that seems quite inappropriate; they can laugh at sad things and cry when there seems to be no cause; they get irritable over trifles, sulky over little things. They weep involuntarily, are worse in the evening and when indoors, better in the open air.

They can also be silently sad and reach a more settled state of depression, despair even, with definite suicidal tendencies. They have impulses to harm themselves, usually with knives but also in other ways. They have violent impulses to stab themselves or to jump from a window. They come to loathe life, to feel that they have had enough of it; they may experience themselves as being completely alone, deserted, separate, worthless. They feel they don't belong, that they have no place in the world, that they are rejected by their god; they get intensely sad and blame themselves.

PULSATILLA NIGRICANS

A *Pulsatilla* depression will reveal the clingy, over-dependent and weepy side of the remedy picture to its maximum. The person will be reluctant to be left alone, full of self-pity, fearful of not being loved, of being abandoned. It may be worse in the morning when she wakes tired and unrefreshed; very discontented, she may weep a long time in the morning. It can also be worse in the evening. She will cry very easily and think everyone is against her, and be very easily hurt. The depression may come about primarily when the person is on her own: there is a desperate fear of abandonment in *Pulsatilla*. It will be accompanied by a terrible indecisiveness, and an enormous need for reassurance and support.

SEPIA

Sepia's symptom picture in depression will be completely withdrawn and melancholy. The person will do nothing but gloom around, occasionally having shouting, rage-filled fits and wanting to leave home. The mood often gets worse as the day goes on and tiredness sets in. The person gets irritable with his family and people close to him, he feels hopeless, worn out, defeated, dragged down. Everything is too much, nothing goes right. He will be very critical and complain constantly, loudly dissatisfied, irritable, quarrelsome and vehement, spiteful and sporadically aggressive with lots of suppressed anger spurting out in uncontrolled outbursts.

He becomes completely indifferent to everything, particularly his partner and family. He feels as if he does not care what happens ('I can't be bothered...' is a common expression). He feels empty inside and is overcome by unaccountable bouts of sadness and involuntary tears. He hides behind a cloud of sepia ink, retiring into a dark moodiness, deliberately cutting himself off from others.

This depression is often precipitated by overwork and adrenal exhaustion. It may also follow viral infection or childbirth, such as in the case of post-natal depression, or in menopausal depression when the typical irritability, fatigue, constipation and backache are nearly always present to some degree.

STAPHYSAGRIA

As with *Natrum muriaticum* you may not observe this type of depression for a while since the person's natural habit is to cover up expression of her feelings. She suppresses everything: anger, indignation, humiliation, grief, and then inevitably becomes chronically resentful and depressed, even suicidally depressed, with deep feelings of worthlessness. She gives up, not caring what happens to her. This depression can be the result of an exhausted nervous system.

STRAMONIUM

This remedy picture may more often show the manic side of the manic-depressive picture, but the depression is also severe. It arises from a deep sense of worthlessness, the person feeling as if he were a piece of wasteland, a garden full of weeds. The depression may alternate with wild and manic behaviour. There will often be some fear discernible in the depression: *Stramonium* is a remedy for great fears. The depression may be strongly influenced by the dark.

The sufferer feels vulnerable to exposure, to injury, to hurt, even looking at himself may be painful. He has a desire to hide, a fear of bright objects and aversion to light, a fear of mirrors, of looking at glass or any reflective object, and of being approached.

SULPHUR

A *Sulphur* depression is characterized by an unshakeable apathy, complete mental and physical burn-out that leaves the person feeling flat. She seems to become very lazy, sitting around doing nothing: she is too lazy to rouse herself and too unhappy to live; she feels tired of life and longs for death. She gets bored, and feels as though she has reached a point where there is nothing left to stimulate her.

Sulphur is very well indicated as a remedy for the seemingly permanent depressed apathy characteristic of some teenagers, when the adolescent falls into a sort of lazy, sullen apathy, staying up all hours and then sleeping long into the next day, losing interest in everything she used to like and becoming absorbed in rather eccentric new interests.

Religious melancholy may be a feature of *Sulphur* depression. The sufferer may be devout but she finds little comfort in her faith and feels anxious about the fate of her soul, relishing religious or existential crises, melancholy, and egocentric brooding.

Sometimes this depression is caused by an overtaxed mind, fatigued by too prolonged or too intense study. The sufferer is apt to feel extremely sorry for herself, feeling so wretched that she would like to die, worrying about the future, becoming hypochondriacal. There is a great tendency to burst into tears.

THUJA OCCIDENTALIS

Depression is strong in the *Thuja* symptom picture – unsurprising considering the extent to which typical *Thuja* personalities suppress and deny their feelings and their deep conviction that there is something wrong and bad about them which needs to be concealed.

Sufferers become stuck in their depressive feelings, thinking that nothing will ever change. They get tired of life, feeling they have had enough of it, and can become suicidal.

Chapter Eight

ANXIETY, PHOBIAS
AND OBSESSIONS

Anxiety is rather a catch-all word, used to describe anything from mild uneasiness and tension through the most acute and terrifying panic attack to persistent, chronic obsessive worries which may destroy a personality.

We live in worrying times, and it is rare to find an adult who does not worry about something. Indeed, it would be worrying to meet such a person! Probably anxiety is to a certain degree healthy: anxiety makes us make preparations for possibilities, makes us check the tyres before going on a long journey, lock the doors at night. A certain amount of nervous tension is necessary for the preservation of life.

However, anxiety and worry only serve a purpose up until they get out of balance and stop us from functioning in the real world. Persistent or excessive anxiety is usually a sign that we need to sort something out, that something is not right in our lives. It's not something simply to be got rid of but something to be understood and then overcome. If we try simply to avoid anxiety without sorting out its real cause then we run the risk of limiting the rest of our lives by concentrating on avoiding people, things and events that cause us anxiety.

Chronic Anxiety and Obsessional Behaviour

The root cause of chronic anxiety and worry is often buried in childhood. We develop certain cautious and self-protective patterns of behaviour at that time, for whatever reason, and then continue to operate out of such patterns long after they are needed. Working with a counsellor may help you to identify the nature and origins of particular patterns of reaction that may no longer be necessary but have become habitual. As a child you may, for instance, have hidden in terror when you heard your parents arguing downstairs: this pattern may have stayed with you on some level so that now you feel terrified of any display of anger, even the merest hint of it. You might feel panicky when you even suspect that someone close to you might be angry. These reactive patterns carry feelings with them from a much earlier time in your life when you were unable to act to solve the problem you faced. Now you may be able to do so.

Obsessional behaviour often forms a strong thread in chronic anxiety. We are all probably obsessional to some degree. We have certain rules by which we keep our lives under control. These rules may seem sensible, even essential to us, and it is often a surprise to realize, for instance, that not everyone has to leave the house completely tidy before leaving for work, not everyone has to straighten all the cushions before going to bed at night, or weigh themselves every morning to make sure not an ounce of extra weight has appeared.

Being obsessed with things means to be completely preoccupied with them, persistently thinking about them. It is often a helpful trait to call on: I would never have finished writing this book, for instance, if I hadn't called on the obsessional part of my personality to think about it constantly and to keep sitting down to it despite the good weather and enticing offers of entertainment. Obsessionally tidy people can be quite an asset in a household: the surfaces are always clean and the vacuuming done. It is when obsessions start interfering with our lives and those of other people that they become a problem.

If we find ourselves checking for burglars in the wardrobes, or repeatedly going back home to check that we have unplugged all the household appliances, threatening divorce if our partner doesn't put a coat away the minute after arriving home, then we should start to think that we might be getting a little obsessional. When we insist that the walls are washed before visitors come to tea, then we're in the grip of a serious obsession.

Real obsessional thoughts are insistent, disruptive and distressing. For instance, a person may be obsessed with knives, constantly preoccupied with thoughts about them. He may, for instance, when seeing one imagine that he could kill himself or his wife or children with it. Anyone can have these impulsive thoughts: usually they just appear, give us a frisson of horror and go. But when compulsion enters into it the person gets the thought repeatedly and can't get free of it. This leads to anxiety about having the thoughts, and fears that the thoughts might be translated into actions. What if he did kill his wife and children? He begins to keep away from knives as much as possible, is afraid to be near them. Some people fear germs like this: They cannot stop thinking about the dangers of contamination, they have to wash their hands at every opportunity, clean the kitchen, even the whole house. Everything has to be scrubbed and disinfected.

Usually we get into such patterns of panic when we are stressed or anxious: we know we are working too hard or not getting enough sleep when we notice that we are obsessively imagining that we will die before we are 50, or when we are insisting that the books on the shelves are colour-coded. Obsessional thoughts are similar in some ways to phobias in that they allow us to focus our attention on a persistent thought or on a ritual activity rather than on the underlying painful feelings.

A common obsessional preoccupation is fear of illness (often cancer): day in, day out you may feel convinced you have cancer. Sometimes this is just a persistent thought that intrudes, other times it has to be acted on – you become convinced and go the rounds of all the doctors looking for a check-up, a diagnosis. Often the originating cause of such an obsession is in some guilt that you feel, justified or not. For instance, the compulsion to worry about one's own death may be an attempt to get rid of the (usually irrational) guilt you feel because someone you were close to or felt responsible for has died (this is known as survivor guilt). Developing the obsessional fear of your own death may replace the process of looking at your own feelings of guilt at being 'responsible' for that person's death.

It is very difficult to change obsessional patterns. The rigid outlook on life which produces such defences as ritual handwashing, cleaning, checking, counting cracks in paving stones remains strong whatever the symptoms, and people with this kind of rigid attitude to life tend to have imposed this degree of limitation and control on their lives for a reason: they will not readily give it up.

Behavioural therapy often works well in removing some of the surface symptoms, but that is probably because it works with the same types of thought structures, with people capable of a disciplined approach and needing a rigid structure. Affirmations may also be helpful with such symptoms, though the substitution of positive affirmations may itself become equally superstitious and obsessional. Some people in our society are addicted to affirmations, but being addicted to good thoughts and a good diet may be preferable to being held in the grip of destructive behaviour.

From what has been said you may be able to imagine which remedies are going to be well indicated for various obsessional patterns: *Anacardium*, *Arsenicum*, *Silica*, *Thuja* are the chief ones.

Acute Anxiety

In some ways acute anxiety is more distressing than chronic anxiety. Many people suffer from distressing and apparently random panic attacks, or particular fears or phobias which to some degree disable them: a fear of open spaces or crowds, for instance.

Panic attacks often seem to come on for no reason. You can be walking down the street, queueing in a store, crossing the street – when suddenly you're terrified, breathing rapidly, getting palpitations, having pains around your heart. Your fingers and toes may be going numb. Or you may wake up in the middle of the night in a panic, startled and aroused and unable to go back to sleep. Your whole nervous system is on red alert. You feel as if you are in shock, that you've just been involved in an accident, a bank robbery, heard some terrible news. These are the symptoms of the well-known fight or flight reaction to threat. They are bad enough when there is a clear, apparent threat, but when they come as if out of the blue for no reason they are incredibly distressing.

What is happening is that your nervous system has become overstressed, either from overwork, poor diet, long continued chronic anxiety or attempting to live in a way you don't like. Your nervous

system starts to go into a flight or fight reaction almost spontaneously, involuntarily. The attack may be triggered by something
that stirs up an unconscious association from the past, a half-
conscious memory, a flash back, a dream or a phobic reaction, for
instance.

Phobias arise as a method of protecting ourselves from other
fears. We allow ourselves (unconsciously) to become afraid of certain
very specific situations or things in order to protect ourselves from
being afraid of or anxious about everything or about some other
particular thing which is altogether too frightening. We collaborate
with our unconscious in order to limit the possibilities for anxiety:
the fear only needs to come on when we are confronted with the
object of fear. Almost anything or any experience can become the
object of phobic fear. The most common phobias focus on being in
high places, going outdoors, being trapped in a small or confining
space, driving in cars or flying, being bitten by animals such as
snakes, bats, dogs, or becoming terminally ill. A phobia can be seen
as a creative attempt by the organism to localize free-floating
anxiety and fear so that we can actually continue our lives. In many
ways it is very efficient to maintain a localized fear of such things as
bats or snakes. These are things which can usually be avoided in life.

However, problems arise when such fears are localized onto
something which cannot be avoided: for example claustrophobia,
which prevents people from using lifts, cars or underground trans-
port systems, or shopping in department stores; or agoraphobia,
which stops people from going outside their houses at all. Even
snakes can be a problem with the increase in natural history
programmes on television.

Unless it has become a serious problem there is something to be
said for leaving phobias alone; they can usually be lived with and are,
in any case, difficult to treat. By the time help is sought most
phobias are entrenched and the original connections to the person's
life are buried out of sight. This is why the treatment most often
advocated in orthodox medicine is behavioural, a method of gradually increasing exposure to the phobia-inducing object until the fear
itself reduces. This may be effective in removing the fear from the
specific object and, if all that remains is the habit of being afraid, the
therapy has a good chance of being successful. If, however, the focus

on one phobia is still serving a useful protective purpose, then either a new object of phobia will emerge or the person may need to be ready to deal with the more free-floating anxiety or with some buried memories.

Many remedies have symptoms of specific phobic reactions, but it is still best to look at the whole picture, using the fact that a specific remedy picture includes a specific phobia as a guide only. Probably the remedies that will work best are the ones that will cover most of the picture whether or not the specific phobia is mentioned. Examples of possible remedies for common phobias are included in the remedy pictures cited below. I have only drawn details from remedies covered by the plan of this book, there are many more remedies with phobic symptoms in their picture.

The most useful remedies in acute anxiety or panic attacks may be *Aconite, Argentum nitricum, Arsenicum, Gelsemium, Ignatia, Stramonium.*

Drugs for Anxiety

Taking drugs for the relief of anxiety may bring about a temporary lessening of symptoms but does nothing to get to the root of why the anxiety arose in the first place, and does not help us to deal with the long-term implications. We have probably all taken such drugs for the relief of anxiety at some time or other, whether prescription drugs, tobacco, alcohol or marijuana. However, all drugs carry potential unpleasant side-effects and tend to be addictive either physically or psychologically, and it is best to avoid them where possible.

The story of the effects of minor tranquillizer prescription in the boom period from the 1960s onwards is as depressing as that of the anti-depressants. Long-term addiction has been the smallest price many anxious people have had to pay for the relief of some of their symptoms. Many others have developed more alarming nerve damage seemingly as a result of taking tranquillizers, the benzodi-azepines in particular. The problems of withdrawal are often worse than the original symptoms: insomnia, palpitations, shakiness, muscle tension, memory loss, anxiety and panic. Though in many cases these symptoms soon pass if the person can be helped through them, in others the withdrawal effects may last for several months and this often leads to the person choosing to go back on the drug rather than endure the withdrawal symptoms. More recently a new group of drugs, similar to those used in depression (such as Prozac and Seroxat), is being used to combat anxiety by raising the level of serotonin in the brain.

All in all it seems best to avoid these where necessary and try to help sort out the problem with homoeopathic remedies. Nearly every remedy picture in the *Materia Medica* includes some degree of anxiety, since it is such a common human experience. The following is a small selection from among the most easily available remedies; if they don't help then consult a homoeopath, who will have access to a wider range of medicines.

Obviously, in any case where anxiety is strong it will be useful to take some other steps to relieve its symptoms: relaxation exercises, perhaps, or listening to relaxation tapes. There is a great variety of these on the market; you will need to find the one that best suits by trial and error. Some people may also be helped by using herbal tranquillizers for a short time. The tissue salt *Kali Phos*, taken daily, is very helpful to many people with jaded nerves; *Avena sativa*, a herbal preparation widely available in health food stores, can also be a long-term support when the person is exhausted due to long-continued anxiety.

ACONITUM NAPELLUS
Useful in panic attacks, acute anxiety, shock or the after-effects of shock, where there is panic, restlessness, shallow breathing, agitation, impatience. There may also be palpitations and sensations of numbness and tingling. The panic may come on for no apparent reason suddenly, often in the evening or at bedtime. The person often has physical symptoms resembling those of a heart attack, and may have strong fears of imminent death, or death at a very exact time. There may also be a fear of suffocation.

Characteristic phobias: air travel, the dark, the dentist, ghosts, agoraphobia and claustrophobia. Having said this, it is worth trying *Aconitum* in any acute situation of fear and panic, whatever the apparent cause.

ANACARDIUM ORIENTALE
The anxiety in this remedy picture emerges from a very low

self-esteem and fear of failure which is masked by a desire to prove oneself and a tough, aggressive, 'hard', even bullying manner.

Intellectually not at all confident, sufferers endure extreme anticipatory anxiety before exams: the mind tends to blank out with exhaustion, the memory is poor in any case and there is an enormous tendency to forget everything, and to become really shaky and nervous before exams.

The typical *Anacardium* state displays two contradictory wills; the person is often in two minds about everything and anything – and this, too, leads to irresolution, indecision, anxiety and inner tension.

Anacardium is also a remedy for many obsessions, all kinds of fixed ideas: that there are demons in the house, that someone is trying to control you, possess you, kill you. Sufferers have fears (often well founded) of going insane, and experience suicidal depressions accompanied by the urge to shoot themselves to stop the voices in their head, to stop the internal torment. They fear that someone has done something to their mind.

ARGENTUM NITRICUM

This remedy picture depicts a person of generally low self-confidence who is afraid of not being able to do whatever it is she sets her mind to do. She is excitable and outgoing, however, and her anxiety will be visible, expressed. She will look agitated, hurried and flustered, worried and apprehensive. She will be 'in a state', trembling with excitement, hot and bothered, often be troubled with nervous diarrhoea, and very much affected by hot atmospheres. She may behave impulsively, always trying to escape from the panicky situation.

She suffers from profound anticipatory anxiety when she has to speak in public, appear on stage, take an exam. She may feel trapped and anxious if she finds herself with a seat in the middle of a row at the theatre, or in a tunnel or a lift. She will be disposed to panic in any situation which she cannot see a way out of, suffer from claustrophobia and agoraphobia, fear of heights, or fear of crowds or a lot of people. She is constantly anxious that something bad will happen. Other specific phobias: air travel, crossing bridges, going to the dentist, health, robbers. She can become tormented by her own thoughts, keep thinking someone is dead, for example, develop superstitious fears – for example that something bad will happen if she doesn't tread on every alternate paving stone. She will be unreasonably anxious if people she loves are even five minutes late home, assuming the worst.

Impulsive behaviour is characteristic: there may be sudden impulses to jump through windows or from high places.

ARSENICUM ALBUM

Arsenicum anxiety is accompanied by extreme restlessness, the person has to be active, moving, doing; he has a driving, worrying, obsessional, workaholic personality that seeks order, structure and control. Critical perfectionists in all they do, sufferers become extremely anxious about falling below their own high standards. Their health is also a great source of worry: they are afraid of serious illness, especially cancer, and they are actively afraid of dying. They are anxious about the possibility of infection or contamination by germs. They are always washing things (especially their hands), and they have an irrational fear of being poisoned.

They are incapable of relaxing, and deal with anxiety by action. Spontaneity and breaking of routine makes them anxious. They will panic if there is not enough time, if things get behind schedule, if their work is disturbed. They are often deeply afraid of their own impulses, of anything spontaneous: they fear harming themselves or others, can't have knives lying around for fear they will use them on someone. They fear some evil, they fear that someone will rob them, they have many fears and anxieties about money. They have a great terror of vomiting, again something that is beyond their control. Naturally, they are afraid of flying.

A very dangerous anxiety state can develop because it can be mixed with depression, despair, weariness of life, suicidal feelings. They will be more anxious when they are alone, when it is dark, and after midnight (particularly between midnight and 3 a.m). In sleep they have anxiety dreams and nightmares: of the dead, of danger, of pursuit.

In acute anxiety and panic attacks the physical symptoms associated with *Arsenicum* are very apparent: the person will be very agitated, probably very short of breath, have palpitations, be restless, need to hurry and walk about, do things. He may also suffer from a paralysing sense of weakness, become quickly prostrated with anxiety or panic. He will need company, will want to hang on to someone, will not be reassured.

AURUM METALLICUM

The personality structure that goes with *Aurum* is extremely conscientious and always anxious to do the right thing, to take responsibilities seriously, to look after people for whom he is responsible. There may be extreme anxiety about having neglected duties and responsibilities, fear of having committed a crime.

Such people are extremely prone to obsessive patterns: they work hard and conscientiously to build something up; identify very strongly with one project or relationship and drive themselves to success, fuelled by a dreadful fear of failure and death. There are great fears of failure, especially the worst failure of all, that they will lose favour with their god.

There is an anxious, obsessive preoccupation with the possibility of getting heart disease and with thoughts of suicide. They fantasize and plan suicide. There is a fear of heights amounting to a phobia, which goes along with an impulse to jump from heights and dreams of falling from them.

The anxiety is restless and agitated and may be accompanied by a restless depressive state, where the sufferer is irascible and self reproaching.

CALCAREA CARBONICA

This symptom picture is one of the most anxious in the *Materia Medica*, second only to that of *Arsenicum*. However, you may not at first realize that a person needing *Calcarea carbonica* is anxious because she is so self-conscious, so concerned about what people will think of her that she covers up any signs of anxiety. She hates being looked at, fearing that she will be laughed at; she is deeply afraid that people will notice what she is 'really' like, that she is crazy, insane. She can become obsessed with the idea that she is going mad and that everyone has noticed it and is looking at her with suspicion.

Many of her anxieties emerge from the fear that she has not enough stamina or strength: she is afraid that she will collapse, won't be able to keep going. She is both agoraphobic and claustrophobic. Other phobias include: flying, disease, insects, mice, rats, snakes, spiders, heights, thunderstorms, insanity, poverty, contamination and germs, the dark, dogs, ghosts, and dentists. This sufferer is also terrified that something evil may happen, of being on her own, and of people. She conceals all this, however, remaining seemingly impassive.

GELSEMIUM SEMPERVIRENS

Gelsemium is a major flu remedy and its characteristic anxiety symptoms can resemble flu symptoms. The things the *Gelsemium* type of person may be anxious about are much the same as those the *Argentum nitricum* personality will be concerned with: anticipatory fears of, for example, being on stage, performing or otherwise appearing in public, air travel, exams, starting school, the dentist. He suffers from fear of public places, agoraphobia, fear of failure, fear that something bad will happen, and thunderstorms. But the way these anxieties will be expressed will be completely opposite to that of *Argentum nitricum*. The sufferer will become utterly low in mind and weak in body, tremulous, slow, sluggish, dull, almost paralysed, wiped out with anxiety. It's a dragging down, tiring anxiety, making the person feel too weak, too frail, too nervous to cope.

As in the picture of *Argentum nitricum* there may be diarrhoea with the anxiety; there may also be problems with vision: blurring or misty vision may be associated with this anxiety.

IGNATIA AMARA

Ignatia is useful for any anxiety state that is expressed in an overexcited way. Think of it as a remedy after any shock or upset when the person is very obviously distressed, but equally trying to control himself (for those people who used to be called 'highly-strung'). He is anxious not to lose control (but does).

This remedy picture depicts a very conscientious, idealistic person, perfectionist, anxious to succeed, suffering from anticipatory anxiety about not being able to do his best. He can be indecisive for fear of making the wrong decision.

The remedy picture is full of anxieties which are largely centred around feelings of being trapped or constricted and being unable to break out. This anxiety is the physical manifestation of the classic *Ignatia* conflict between a person's perception of the ideal and reality. Specific fears: of cancer, closed places, being poisoned, robbers.

LACHESIS

The *Lachesis* remedy picture represents a state of pent-up nervous and sexual energy which has to be expressed: if it cannot be then there is intense anxiety and restlessness.

This anxiety is often unbearable on waking, and on going to sleep; there is a lot of anxiety about the future as well as many sexual anxieties and jealousies.

In the *Lachesis* state a person is fundamentally suspicious and has many intense fears arising from this: that someone is going to come into her house and steal something, of being poisoned, that people will hurt her, of almost anyone (paranoia), of imminent death. She also fears germs and contamination, snakes, dogs and thunderstorms. Delusions of persecution can develop and you may notice that she is in a state of severe paranoia. In this state the sufferer may fear being possessed, have delusions that people will kill her, hear voices telling her to kill or to confess to crimes she has not committed, or be convinced that God will punish her.

LYCOPODIUM CLAVATUM

This is one of the broadest and deepest-acting of all the remedies indicated for anxiety.

The person needing *Lycopodium* suffers from a lack of self-confidence and a chronic fear of failure which is well masked by his air of competence and authority. Whenever anything is going to happen which may lead to not being able to keep up this front he is very anxious, hence he suffers from extreme anticipatory anxiety before public speaking, exams, performance of any kind. He will over-prepare, then perform very well or achieve excellent results, but will still feel inadequate and lack self-confidence. Fear of change and of anything new is also marked, and for the same reason: the sufferer doubts his ability. He learns to avoid new situations in order to evade the panic that accompanies them.

He may have panic attacks, get into states of mental confusion, become unable to make decisions. He suffers from many fears: excessive concern about his health and financial security, fear of crowds, of crossing bridges, of closed places, the dark, death, ghosts, insects, thunderstorms, dining out in public, going out of the house, not being able to achieve what he has set out to do, of impotence (and impotence through fear), and of the opposite sex.

This anxiety can become obsessional and result in trembling fear, insomnia, collapse and exhaustion.

NATRUM MURIATICUM
This is the remedy for the person who conceals anxiety very well, in this case in order to avoid the sympathy and concern of others at all costs. Her anxiety is provoked by anything which threatens change in her routine: weekend visitors even. It is not always concealed: in a situation of acute anxiety there may be an *Ignatia*-like reaction with sudden swings between tears and laughter.

Agoraphobia is a problem, there is also claustrophobia. The person is already closed off, and anything that makes her feel more so is seen as a threat. Phobias include: fear of robbers, of the house being broken into, of being poisoned, of flying, of the dark, of dogs, of insects (especially bumble bees and spiders), and of thunderstorms; fear of heights, of loss of control; fear of being ridiculed or laughed at; a great fear of illness, hypochondria.

NUX VOMICA
The person who needs this remedy is in a permanent state of anxiety and nervous tension. He makes unrealistic demands on himself all the time and tries to reach impossible standards. The anxiety is likely to be accompanied by short-temperedness. He deals with his tension by working harder and harder, and gets bored and depressed if he can't work. He has sexual insecurities and anxieties too. He is apprehensive about work, the future, his physical safety, financial security, health (less acutely than in the case of an *Arsenicum* anxiety).

PHOSPHORUS
The anxiety in this remedy picture arises from being over-impressionable, over-sensitive to the environment. Sufferers are

strongly affected by all sorts of external stimuli: changes in the weather, storms, light, noise. They are also full of fears: the dark, deep water, dogs, death, being alone, being robbed, all cause terror. They also fear that something dreadful will happen, that someone will die. They are extremely nervous and sensitive, worse at twilight, afraid of ghosts, and worse for music and thunder. They sense negative forces in the atmosphere. They are anxious about their health, imagining they have every disease they read or hear about, especially cancer. They are afraid of being poisoned.

Sufferers are prone to panic attacks and can experience sensations of numbness and shakiness, heart palpitations, and the strange feeling that they are leaving their bodies. They seek reassurance, but can be (unlike, for example, someone who needs *Arsenicum*) reassured.

PLATINUM METALLICUM

This remedy picture depicts a state of great insecurity and despair masked by an air of haughtiness and pride. Sufferers are full of fears and anxieties, they fear that something terrible will happen (for instance that their partner or children will not come home). They fear violent death: they fear being strangled, murdered, being hanged. Physical illnesses may come on after fright.

They have other anxieties: about their health (fear of heart disease, fear of having a stroke) and as a result of joyful things or excitement. This anxiety is often felt in the heart, with palpitations. They may have premonitions about dying, and fear imminent death and imaginary forms (ghosts). When anxious they tend to be restless and excitable, walking about, trembling, with breathing difficulties and violent palpitations. They can suffer from agoraphobia, fear of dogs, or a fear of knives.

PULSATILLA NIGRICANS

This remedy is indicated for nervous, timid people who need a lot of reassurance. They will suffer from claustrophobia in stuffy rooms, will fear being alone, and the dark, and ghosts (in the evening), and crowds. They are likely to be irritable when anxious. They are anxious about whether other people approve of them. *Pulsatilla* anxiety is of an irritable, peeved type in a personality that is outwardly passive and apparently easily led.

In acute anxiety the person is likely to show the typical *Pulsatilla* symptoms of sensitivity to warm atmospheres and stuffy environments: 'I have to get out, get some fresh air,' claustrophobic sensations.

The major fear in *Pulsatilla* is of being abandoned; everything revolves round this. The whole personality has developed in such a way as to protect itself against this possibility.

Specific phobias include: fear of open places, public places, of crossing bridges, of closed places, of the dark, of dogs, of ghosts.

SILICA

The person needing *Silica* is timid and anxious generally, insecure and indecisive yet obstinate and even obsessional. She is anxious about whether she can do what she is supposed to do, whether she can last, whether she has the necessary stamina. She is preoccupied with the possibility of failure. Such a person may be physically weak or have a history of not having been well in childhood. Her lack of confidence tends to stem from this actual physical weakness. *Silica* is thus a remedy for long-standing obsessional states where weakness and exhaustion are marked.

Sufferers feel completely inadequate and this makes them focus on very small things, on the detail at the expense of the big picture. They are conscientious about trifles and will sit and count pins or other small objects. They are afraid to undertake anything for fear they will fail. They can become quite obsessional, obstinate and self-willed, all out of their fear of failure. They have an obsessional conviction of their own inadequacy which can be quite paralysing. They are dominated by fear and weakness, and by fixed ideas of their own weakness.

Specific phobias: dogs, exams, appearing in public, robbers, thunderstorms.

STRAMONIUM

Stramonium is useful when anxiety has reached panic levels, when the fear comes on suddenly in a wild frenzy, such as that brought on by sudden shock, fright, high fever, or physical injury.

This anxiety is characterized by an extreme fear of the dark, of being alone, of tunnels or any closed narrow places, of animals (especially dogs), of being devoured by animals, of shining expanses of water, of ghosts and cemeteries, of being murdered. Night terrors are strong. The child wakes screaming, terrified, and doesn't recognize his parents. The fears are intense and violent and there will be a violent reaction to them: cursing, shouting, smashing things, and possibly other violent behaviour.

SULPHUR
Sulphur's anxiety may be concealed beneath an air of self-assurance: the person talks a lot, and seems to know everything. However, he is anxious quite a lot of the time, especially when he is alone in bed and when contemplating the future. He can become anxious about a whole range of moral and religious questions, and about the possibility of catching diseases. When ill he can be quite fussy and picky, reminiscent of the *Arsenicum* type of remedy picture.

He is apprehensive about the future, wherein he sees nothing but misery and suffering; he is apprehensive about the safety of others (because of his over-imagination, not out of any genuine concern for them).

Specific fears: closed places, contamination, germs, dogs, heights, thunderstorms.

THUJA OCCIDENTALIS
This remedy picture probably covers the greatest range of obsessional symptoms (fixed ideas) in the *Materia Medica*, even more than *Arsenicum* or *Silica*. The inflexibility of sufferers is extensive. People who need this remedy have the most fixed ideas, the most rigid thought patterns. They are extremely anxious about many things: the approach of strangers, their desire to be alone, about foreign bodies in their food, about cancer or some other illness. They mull over their past failures, feel they have committed a crime, worry about the future and are fearful of their salvation. They are very scrupulous over little things and touchy over trivial matters as well. Their minds are preoccupied with persistent ideas. They get stuck in one track and find it difficult to get off it. They have fears of going mad, of losing control, of leaving their bodies.

When their obsessiveness gets to a pathological level sufferers may become convinced that someone is following them; they may hallucinate that a stranger is sitting beside them, or that their body and soul have separated, or that they are made of glass and will break. They may develop fixed ideas about being under the influence of a super-human power. They may have delusions about demons and spirits trying to control their minds. They feel that someone is trying to possess them or trying to manipulate their minds to make them do things they do not want to do. They fear losing control, and going insane.

Specific fears: contamination, germs, strangers.

Chapter Nine

THE EFFECTS OF CHILD ABUSE

The subject of child abuse in general and child sexual abuse in particular has been talked about and studied intensively over the last few years, having been substantially ignored and actively denied for many more years previously. We are beginning to realize, with horror, that abuse of children, whether sexual, physical or psychological, is far more widespread than had been realized. We are confronted daily in newspapers and on television with contemporary evidence of how cruel adults can be to children, and how sexually invasive and abusive. Many women have had some sort of abusive encounter with an adult before they reach puberty, and this may also be true for more men than currently reveal or recall what has happened to them.

When Sigmund Freud, the founder of modern psychological theory, saw his first clients at the end of the nineteenth century, he discovered that many of their problems appeared to have originated in sexual abuse in childhood. The implications of this discovery so disturbed him that he actually left the evidence out of the published versions of his case notes, and founded his whole psychological system on a perhaps more comfortable theory: that the patients were fantasizing that they had had sexual relations with their fathers, mothers, uncles. We now seem to be rediscovering what Freud already knew but could not allow himself to make public.

Now, at the end of the twentieth century, many people are recovering memories of having been sexually abused as children. The memories return in fragmentary form, in half-remembered glimpses and recollections of bodily sensations that seem inappropriate to our adult selves, in flashbacks, and in sudden vivid images which return at all sorts of times: when making love, when walking idly through woods. Incidents which have been forgotten and walled off because the childhood psyche was unable to deal with them at the time filter back to consciousness in this way. This is not surprising: it is agreed by all psychotherapists that 'forgetting' in this way is one of the standard means by which children (and adults) deal with traumatic events which are too much for them.

To give a simple example of the process: a few years ago I was walking in the country with a friend when we came across some donkeys, one of whom mistook my thumb for a carrot and tried to gobble it up. I was frankly terrified, but fortunately my friend eventually persuaded the donkey to let me go. The thumb healed and I forgot the incident. At a much later date I developed pains in this thumb – sharp, shooting pains which mystified me: I couldn't remember having done anything to it. Then one night I was watching a natural history programme on TV when the presenter rested his hand on the jaw of a horse's skeleton to make some point: I, sitting peacefully in my armchair, broke out into a violent sweat, couldn't breathe, went into a panic attack, and at the same time had a total recall of the incident with the donkey. I calmed myself down, the pains went away and never came back. This is a simple example of the process which takes place after any trauma. I, of course, was able to check my memory with my friend in a way that people who remember sexual abuse as children cannot.

When children are abused they may 'forget' what happened in the way described above, and may get similar panic attacks, flashbacks, when exposed to apparently neutral events which remind them, on some deep level, of what happened to them as children. The forgetting may also be accompanied by a number of other processes. Children may develop certain personality structures to defend against what has happened to them, for example a tough or placatory attitude to their abuser, or they may split off their knowledge of what happened, containing it within a separate little personality. Nothing happened to them, it happened to 'Gloria'. Such personality attitudes developed in childhood to protect against invasion may later inhibit the development of an integrated adult life, or perhaps these memories may start to come back, threatening to overturn the already fragile personality structures developed in response to the original trauma.

Working with the effects of child abuse in adults involves helping people to deal with very disturbing material at the time when memories may begin to come back, helping them respond to the frightening half-memories and flashbacks. It also involves supporting someone in the process of deconstructing a personality which has been built up in response to abuse, at the time when the person wishes to reorganize and live in response to life in the present, not the past.

Being with or working with someone who is in the process of recovering memories of abuse of any kind, but particularly of sexual abuse, is a very delicate process and should in no way be forced. Only the person involved knows what has happened and there should be no prompting or suggestions made. It should never be suggested that abuse is at the root of current problems even if this seems obvious to you. If it is there and it is important for the person to know it, it will come through. People must be allowed to recover the memories in their own way and in their own time.

All cruel treatment, physical or emotional, all sexual assault, all trauma, leaves lasting and painful effects, but the effects of abuse on children are particularly long-lasting precisely because they are created at a time when we are trying to form a working personality structure to last us for seventy-odd years. To be abused as a child is to be undermined and hurt when at one's most vulnerable and defenceless, more, to be undermined by those who purport to be our protectors, to have gross interference in the normal process of forming the personality at the time most crucial to that process. What started out in childhood as temporary strategies to deal with an intolerable situation seem to become fixed parts of the adult personality, no longer necessary (perhaps) but rigidly embedded in that original fear.

There is no real way to measure the effects of child abuse on any one given child. Abuse can range from being screamed at in the supermarket to being subject to sustained sexual abuse, and its apparent repercussions can range from shyness in company to actual psychosis. Though some forms of abuse may seem worse than others, in fact the effects are not necessarily proportionate to the apparent severity or outrageousness of the abuse. Many children have suffered terribly from apparently small acts of careless cruelty or neglect, others have escaped fairly intact from what seem to be horrific situations. We do not know the reason for the differing effects, unless it is the nature of the child's original constitution, or the nature of the whole relationship between child and parents, child and significant others.

Nor do we know what makes the difference in recovery from childhood abuse. For some people, as the memories return and are dealt with, so the events of the past recede and take their place as part of the whole of life; the personality can be reformed once the origins of some of the distortions can be understood and accepted. Others seem to get 'stuck' and find themselves unable to move on from the point of identifying themselves as survivors of sexual abuse. This is in no way a criticism or a judgment, merely an observation. We all get stuck in our past patterns, whatever their origin. It is my hope that a wider knowledge about the possibility of using homoeo-pathic remedies for the effects of child abuse will enable more people to move on. I am not naïve enough to think that these severe consequences can be 'cured' merely by a remedy, but I do know that the energy, the emotional charge around them can be beneficially affected by a remedy.

I am not going to talk here in any detail about dealing with the direct effects of current abuse on a child. This is a matter for immediate action by concerned adults. However, it should be remembered that when children are abused, sexually harassed, or frightened, the effects initially are similar to those of shock, and the remedies which may be useful at the time will be those that help with shock and injury that results from any assault: *Arnica*, *Aconite* and *Staphysagria* would be the main ones indicated here. Remedies may also be used to help with the physical effects of abuse: *Arnica*, *Staphysagria*, *Bellis Perennis*, or *Echinacea* may be needed.

In order to present a picture (albeit short and sketchy) of some of the characteristic effects on the adult personality of child abuse, I am going to describe the well-chronicled and well-established consequences of long-term constant physical or sexual abuse. This will provide a fuller picture of the potential effects of child abuse on the adult, and of the strategies developed over time by young people who have suffered from such abuse. In fact these strategies are very little different from the strategies we have all learned to use, whether we are aware of having been abused or not, to protect ourselves from the feelings of terror and out-of-controlness that are actually part and parcel of being children, helpless in an adult world.

As already mentioned above, many people forget that they have been abused as children. They repress the awful memories and live in ignorance of the facts, often unaware of what has happened to them. The memories may start to come back in later life, trickling or flooding through and causing great confusion. There may be flashbacks to scenes of the original abuse, there may be 'body memories' without actual images or words. There may be panic attacks, or physical illnesses of unexplained nature. There may be sudden hatred of once-loved people, or overreactions to certain smells or sights. At this time remedies such as *Aconite* may be helpful in calming the fear and making sense of the confusion.

How could anyone possibly forget having been abused, especially having been so horrifically abused as some accounts indicate? Because it is *essential for survival* at the time to forget. A child needs to be able to trust the people who care for her. If she cannot, if she is being neglected, attacked or sexually assaulted by her carers, she has to develop strategies to preserve her relationship with them: she may, for instance, deny, even to herself, that it is happening; she may lie to others about her relationship with her parents, pretending it is marvellous and that she is special to them. Or she may take another line, convincing herself that she is wicked and deserves what is happening to her. Many children do both, in order to preserve the idea that their parents (or at least one of them) are good and trustworthy in the face of daily evidence of their malice, helplessness or indifference. The child alters the unbearable reality in her mind when she is unable to alter it in fact.

If she denies that it is happening she learns to dissociate from it. She learns to leave her body, 'zoom out', go away – go, often, into a kind of trance. She does this both while it is happening, so as not to feel the pain, and then after it has happened, to pretend it has never occurred. Children who are bullied at school often do this, too. In this way they can ignore severe pain, forget whole tracts of experience, develop a completely altered sense of time and place – anything to protect themselves from knowing what happened. Though they may be deliberate at the outset, these alterations of consciousness often become automatic and involuntary.

In adult life what started out as a temporary strategy can become very troublesome. The disowned and dissociated feelings may lie there walled off but waiting to explode. They may return in later life in puzzling 'overreactions' to violence, to particular scenes in films, to particular sexual acts, to certain social situations. The now grown-up person may feel fear or anxiety in particular situations but be unable to account for it. Dining out in public may become difficult. Thus phobias and obsessions often originate in childhood as attempts to control and limit fears of annihilation.

This dissociation may have been so complete as to have involved the creation of completely separate personalities with their own names, functions and memories. The child creates these other personalities, known these days as 'alters', to make it possible for her to cope with the abuse by keeping it outside of her ordinary awareness. It didn't happen to me, it happened to 'Jane'. The adult isn't in touch with any of the feelings that Jane had.

The dissociation may have been so powerful that the sufferer becomes unable to feel anything at all, going through life dissociating habitually from emotion. In some cases she may discover that she can bring herself back, get out of this state of dissociation by cutting or stabbing or hurting herself in some way. Physical pain is much preferable to the emotional pain that it replaces, and it also proves the existence of the survivor. Self-injury is not intended to kill, it is not a suicidal gesture, but it is designed to relieve unbearable emotional pain. It is also a way of turning the anger she feels against her abuser inwards, towards herself, an expression of self-hatred often directed at specific areas of the body which are a source of shame for her. Self-injury is only the most spectacular of the many ways in which abused children discover that they can alter their emotional state, can 'bring themselves back': other ways include purging and vomiting, compulsive sexual behaviour, compulsive risk-taking and drug abuse. These self-destructive symptoms are often well established in abused children even before adolescence; they become much more prominent in the adolescent years, and often continue into adulthood. Here remedies such as *Arsenicum*, *Lachesis*, *Platina* or *Staphysagria* may be helpful.

Another strategy that is often used is that the child constructs some system of meaning that justifies the abuse, usually adopting the explanation that she is wicked, evil. Since this is an explanation often freely offered by the abusing parent in any case, the child does not have to look far to find it. The advantage to the child is that it gives her some control in the situation. If it is her fault that these terrible things are happening to her, then she can do something about it. She can stop being wicked, she can be good, she can do whatever the abuser wants, she can placate, please. She can easily convince herself that her rage and murderous feelings (natural responses to abuse) are evidence of her wickedness. Likewise, if she is sexually aroused or gets some physical excitement during the abuse this is further proof of her evil: it proves that she really does want it, she really is wicked, she does deserve it. She can punish herself to assuage her feelings of guilt.

If, as children, we have adopted the line of defence that we are wicked, this remains with us as adults. We may continue to feel that there is something really wrong with us, something twisted and not to be seen or else people will hate us. We may feel that we have committed the unforgivable sin, that we are deeply and unchangeably wicked, dirty and untrustworthy. Our self-contempt can be profound. We have built up the core of our identity around this unshakeable fact, that we are wicked, and we may live in fear of anyone discovering what we are really like, perhaps avoiding meaningful relationships for fear of being found out, seen through.

Both as children and as adults, however, we try to be 'good'. We can become superb over-achievers, at school, in the kitchen, wonderful at looking after our parents, doing things for them, perfectionist in all things. We can take control of our own lives this way, always doing things right before anyone can criticize or punish us, or, anticipating blame, we can apologize for our very existence. We can become very practised at noticing danger signals, at noticing when things are not quite right. We may become very good at what we do in adult life as a result of our early survival training, but we always feel this successful self to be inauthentic, false. If people appreciate us we simply have it confirmed that no one really knows us and that, if they did know us – if our true selves were revealed – we would be hated.

The effects of child abuse are, in fact, now recognized as a special case of post-traumatic stress disorder (PTSD), the modern term for the condition which often results when people have been involved in any traumatic situation: sexual assault, rape, violent robbery or assault, war, being taken hostage or sent to a concentration camp, witnessing a murder, being involved in a serious accident or natural disaster, living in inner-city areas frequented by violent gangs or terrorists. In these conditions the fear of injury, loss of life or annihilation produces complex effects.

The author Judith Herman Lewis (see *Further Reading*, Appendix One) has proposed that child abuse be included in the category 'complex post-traumatic stress disorder', comparable with the effects of having been a hostage for a long time, for instance, because it is not only the shock but the impossibility of escaping from the situation that makes it necessary to construct so many false selves.

People suffering from PTSD in general suffer from a persistent re-experiencing of the trauma (through nightmares, flashbacks, re-stimulation by similar events), a great need to avoid anything remotely resembling the stress, and signs of 'increased arousal' (insomnia, irritability, difficulty concentrating, fearfulness, physical signs of anxiety). They feel all sorts of emotions: guilt and shame, terrible anxiety. This is what happens also for survivors of child abuse. Where the abuse has been sexual then clearly there may be complications in sexual relationships, or physical complications in sexual areas of the body. A new event in the individual's life, such as getting married or having a baby, may re-stimulate the stress reaction from childhood, often without the individual being able to remember the earlier traumatic event. Some experts believe that childhood sexual abuse always leads to PTSD in adulthood.

There is another issue which needs to be addressed here, that of the so-called False Memory Syndrome. As increasing numbers of adults have remembered being abused as children, so many have confronted their abusers (in cases where they are still alive) as part of their own healing process. The accused have normally denied the accusations. As a result the idea of False Memory Syndrome has been brought forward: it is suggested that many, if not all, such memories are false, hysterical, and that they have been implanted in the person's mind while under hypnosis. Some accused parents have formed pressure groups, False Memory Syndrome organizations, to challenge the belief that memories of sexual abuse are accurate. Therapists are being accused of encouraging false memories, and the adults who are remembering childhood abuse are again being put into the position of not being allowed to speak their truth. It is obviously important that parents should not be falsely accused, or left without redress. But high-profile court cases may have the effect of stifling the free expression of memories of abuse.

People remember sexual abuse in different ways, all of which may be subject to other interpretations: there may be 'body memories' actual memories, flashbacks, dreams or images which come while in a trance state, either self-induced or occurring while under hypnosis. It is important to recognize that anyone who gets memories and flashbacks of having been abused as a child has definitely felt *abused* in some way. This does not mean that the abuse occurred precisely as 'remembered'. It is well known that even only a short time after any event has taken place, each of the people present will remember completely different things. It is also well known that in areas or topics other than sexual abuse, the unconscious mind uses all sorts of imagery and metaphor to communicate material and information to the conscious present. Why should this not be the case in matters of abuse? There may even be a difference between a 'memory' and a dream or a flashback. What seems to be remembered may be a very accurate and literal representation of what happened, or it may be, to varying degrees, a metaphorical representation of what happened. We cannot be clear.

However, the child's experience clearly was that she was attacked, invaded, trespassed on, treated cruelly. Her unconscious may communicate this to her in images of physical attack or sexual penetration which may not be literally accurate – however, the feelings represent a truth which needs to emerge in order for progress to be made. The feeling and the response to those feelings are what underlie the various personality difficulties which exist in the present.

I am not saying that people who remember that they were abused as children were not so abused. Undoubtedly many of the people who remember abuse have been abused in precisely the way that they remember, and there is plenty of evidence all around us that the abuse of children is widespread. For others, however, the language of abuse may be the language of metaphor, a way to explain an abuse of an equally terrifying though less material nature. We must not lose sight of this important fact in the process of trying to be legally accurate and to protect the accused parent, where innocent. The child in the adult must continue to be protected as well.

To have been abused as a child is to have been hurt when at one's most vulnerable and defenceless: the effects are to bring into existence defensive personality structures, which differ according to the existing constitutional structure of each person. It is these structures which are addressed by homoeopathic remedies.

Almost all, if not all of the conditions described in this book will have had their origins in childhood, since that is where, powerless, we all first learned to deal with crises in ways which later prove to be inappropriate and destructive to our adult life and to interfere with our best mode of functioning. The protective devices adopted by survivors of child abuse are not different in kind from those adopted by all children trying simply to survive to adulthood, although they may be different in degree. However, we can all change these maladaptations when they are no longer necessary to us, and this is where homoeopathic remedies can come in, along with other ways of facilitating change.

There are no 'remedies for child abuse'; all abused children have reacted in their own individual ways to what has happened to them. Any remedy which matches the personality of the person concerned may be of help to someone who has been abused as a child, because the remedy chosen on this basis will match what remains as the chief defensive mechanism erected. However, it can be seen that a number of remedy pictures appear more frequently than others to match some of the more common symptom pictures of child abuse and of PTSD generally. In the following descriptions attention will be drawn to such features, as well as to some of the characteristic defensive structures.

ACONITUM NAPELLUS
This is, of course, a most important remedy for shock both in the immediate moment of the first experience and years afterwards,

when the effects of the original shock may begin to resurface. It is perhaps the best remedy for simple post-traumatic stress disorder, and for panic attacks of unknown origin.

ANACARDIUM ORIENTALE

The *Anacardium* picture cries out as that of someone who has been abused as a child. All the essential elements are there: extremely low self-esteem, a mixture of meekness and submissiveness with anger and violence.

This remedy picture is one of several which portrays in a marked way the 'splitting off' mentioned above. The major split may be between the felt 'good' and 'evil' parts of the person, expressed by the sense he or she may have of having an angel on one shoulder, a devil on the other, and the way in which such types flip between the two behaviours, sometimes apparently involuntarily or compulsively. This split is sometimes seen as one between the meek and the malicious, the placator and the abuser, the submissive and the bully, a split often seen in those who have been forced to submit to abuse and humiliation.

The remedy picture also depicts sensations of splitting off from the body, common in those who have been abused or badly frightened. It also includes all kinds of fixed ideas suggestive of the fact that the person has been invaded as a child: that there are demons in the house, that someone is trying to possess or even to kill him; sensations that someone is trying to control his mind, or that mind and body are separate, or that the soul is leaving the body.

ARSENICUM ALBUM

The *Arsenicum* personality structure could very well have emerged from a traumatic childhood. The often extreme desire for control and orderliness, the over-achieving perfectionism, the desire to be good are all diagnostic factors. The basic insecurity of *Arsenicum* has been attributed to fear of abandonment, which is certainly what happens to the abused child. The *Arsenicum* obsessional state has clearly evolved in order to protect against anything unexpected happening. Children check under beds, tidy everything, collect litter. Their obsessive tidiness is designed to impose some order over a hostile environment. Fastidiousness and fear of contamination, strong elements in the *Arsenicum* picture, are also often associated with the repression of sexual memories.

Arsenicum is also highly indicated in anorexia and self-mutilating behaviour, often found where there is a history of childhood sexual abuse. The remedy picture includes constant fantasies of cutting the body with a knife or razor blade, and thoughts of self-mutilation. This usually represents an impulse to cut rather than to kill. There is a corresponding fear of knives and a desire to strike the head and the person. Anxiety is worse at night.

LYCOPODIUM CLAVATUM

Lycopodium presents a picture of someone who may have been extensively abused as a child, though not necessarily sexually (more likely emotionally). *Lycopodium* appears to have been bullied and put down dreadfully. It may be because of this that we see the assumed air of superiority, the careful concentration on an area of expertise in which the person can take control, become an expert, as well as the constant underlying fear of exposure, the terrible desire to get it right, to placate and please others even while hiding behind a shield of haughtiness. This behaviour pattern may be the product of an early life spent with a domineering parent.

NATRUM MURIATICUM

This is obviously a remedy which will be useful for someone who has built a wall around her over a period of many years so that no one is allowed to pass her boundaries. The origin of such a walled defence may well lie in the experiences of 'boundary crossing' in childhood, of having had to endure repeated invasions of personal space and privacy. The *Natrum muriaticum* defence system has been designed to repel all intruders, to regard any approach as a potential robbery.

Included in the *Natrum muriaticum* picture will be grief at the loss of the loved and trusted person, at the breach of trust. The *Natrum muriaticum* attachment to the past can be a serious block to recovery. She is haunted by unpleasant thoughts about the past, about how she has been wronged; she bears grudges against anyone who has offended her. It may be difficult for someone with this personality structure to break the mould.

PLATINUM METALLICUM

Platina is clearly a remedy well indicated for the long-lasting effects of child sexual abuse. Here we see the creation of the superior self, a 'special' person who is more desirable, more attractive, more important than others, reflected in the attitudes of superiority and haughtiness which are an integral part of the *Platina* personality structure. We also see the opposite feelings of utter worthlessness and suicidal depression.

That the abuse was probably sexual is suggested by the high level of symptoms, both emotional and physical, connected with the sexual and genital areas. There is a lot of conflict and difficulty surrounding this person's strong sex drive – *Platina* does not simply enjoy sex, as does the *Phosphorus* type, she has to have it. In *Platina* there is always conflict about sexuality as well.

In the physical sphere there are a lot of symptoms associated with the sexual system in women. There are painful periods, ovarian pain, vaginismus, compulsive masturbation during sleep, and great sensitivity around the vulval and vaginal areas. The genital area seems extremely sensitive to touch; there is also a tendency to itching and irritation, numbness and tingling sensations. This can be either pleasurable or uncomfortable. It may encourage sexual desire or make sexual intercourse uncomfortable, even impossible. There may be excessive or compulsive masturbation in children.

Add to this the heightened and often precocious awareness of sexual matters, and the extreme jealousy and insecurity that accompanies sexual relationships. *Platina* may be a useful remedy where people feel driven to sexual promiscuity. On the other hand it may be useful for people whose sex drive has been suppressed. Sexuality, like other aspects of the *Platina* picture, is prone to be exaggerated or distorted.

The *Platina* personality is, in short, sexually very excitable, easily aroused, and may be obsessed with sexual activity. Her sleep may be interrupted by disturbing sexual dreams. If psychosis supervenes there is a hugely sexual content in the delusions, and she may talk constantly of sexual matters.

Dissociation is part of the *Platina* remedy picture, and so is the formation of multiple personalities. Familiar objects may appear strange and different. Those affected wake in the middle of the night with feelings of having left their body.

PULSATILLA NIGRICANS

Pulsatilla is not usually identified as a remedy for the effects of child abuse, child sexual abuse anyway, but it can readily be seen that the *Pulsatilla* mode of remaining childlike, appealing to others for support and help, is strongly conciliatory. *Pulsatilla* always tries to find out how to please those who have power over him, adopting the hostage-conciliator mode. *Pulsatilla* is thus a remedy for any person who feels himself powerless for whatever reason and has learned to use dependency and helplessness rather than outright aggression as a means of getting the support he needs. It is the complete picture of the victim sub-personality. *Pulsatilla* also has a fear of the opposite sex in its picture. Likewise it has many difficulties centred around food and eating, often an issue for those who have been sexually abused (see Chapter Ten).

STAPHYSAGRIA

This is the major remedy to be considered where there has been specifically sexual abuse in childhood and the child has dealt with it initially by forgetting about it, remembering only part of it, or remembering it and blaming herself. When the adult begins to re-examine that part of her life, either by allowing memories to come back or by allowing herself to get angry, this may be the time for *Staphysagria*.

Staphysagria is characterized by suppressed indignation and resentment and pent-up anger. The person feels it is her fault; she feels guilty. She feels she is a bad person, dirty and unclean, that she has done something wicked. The *Staphysagria* personality has adopted the defence of being sweet and humble and passive. She tries to do everything just right for everyone because of her fear of being punished, of being shouted at. She learns to give in.

The *Staphysagria* remedy picture often includes a history of being humiliated or hurt in other than sexual ways. It is the main remedy for children who have been physically abused (beaten up or hit) and emotionally humiliated.

Accompanying symptoms include a distortion of the body image, as in anorexia. There may be self-harm. Obsessional sexual ideas which are extremely disturbing may develop. There is often a history of high sexual desire and a lot of relationships.

STRAMONIUM

This may be one of the most commonly indicated remedies for the effects of child abuse. When you think of the number of fears and terrors and anxieties associated with the dark and the night, the reasons will be obvious. The second element which might make it well indicated would be its very strong sexuality, the sexualization that comes of much experience. The deep sense of worthlessness frequently seen in *Stramonium* may also point in this direction, as does the impulsive and violent behaviour, the effects of long split-off rage.

THUJA OCCIDENTALIS

Sexual and physical abuse clearly may have played their part in the development of the *Thuja* defence mechanism. A person who needs *Thuja* is prone to feel that there is something unusual about his sexuality and his feelings, but he keeps quiet about it: this is one of the biggest keynotes. The person who needs *Thuja* may have secret sexual desires or fantasies and may masturbate secretly. He is ashamed of and secretive about these habits, which is not necessarily the case for other types of people in many cultures today. A major cause of the *Thuja* secretiveness, the feeling that he is at bottom bad and must pretend to be nice, may be the result of sexual abuse in childhood. The splitting-off that is inherent in the remedy picture may have been necessary then.

What the sufferer fears is that others will find out that he has done something wrong, bad, fundamentally unacceptable. Thus he keeps things to himself, concealing both his feelings and his thoughts, presenting the world with a different image of himself from what he really feels himself to be. He closes down his feelings, believing that they are somehow unacceptable. He may have a sense of being separate (which he is), feeling as if he were divided into two parts, that his mind and body are separated. He splits off from his feelings. He loses touch with his physical self as part of this splitting-off process. His bodily sensations may feel strange, he may describe feeling as if his soul is separated from his body, that one half of him is alienated from the other, that there is something moving around inside him (in women sufferers this can manifest as a conviction or fear that they are pregnant).

Chapter Ten

EATING DISORDERS

The best-known and probably most common type of obsessional behaviour current in our society at the moment is that connected with food and body image. Many people are obsessional about the way they look and what they eat, and go to enormous lengths to control their weight and shape by diet and exercise. At any given time more than 80 per cent of women are depriving themselves of food for one reason or another, and it is estimated that one in four of the population will suffer from some sort of eating disorder in their lives.

These figures represent only the tip of an iceberg of huge proportions, for almost everyone has or has had at some time, problems about self-image, weight and body size. We nearly all feel 'too thin' or 'too fat', never 'just right'. We nearly all eat for comfort or starve for fashion, only a matter of degree separating the mass of half-hearted dieters from those people who diet, run, go to the gym and obsess about their body shape and calorie intake, and only a further matter of degree separating these people from those who fall into the more extreme behaviours of the recognized eating disorders: anorexia, bulimia and compulsive eating. The prevalence of these conditions has almost doubled in the last 20 years (or perhaps the correct diagnosis is now being made more often). Alarmingly, young children are now being diagnosed as suffering from eating disorders, so strong is society's message that we should be a certain shape and size.

In anorexia the woman wants to be as thin as possible, so is concerned to limit her food intake to the barest minimum: she rejects food, becomes preoccupied with methods of refusing it, disguising the fact that she is not eating, employing some bingeing and vomiting to get rid of what little she does eat. She is permanently preoccupied with losing weight, always considering herself to be too fat even when she is nothing but skin and bone.

In bulimia the woman is just as anxious to be thin but adopts different methods to achieve her end, usually overeating in binges and then taking laxatives or making herself sick to get rid of the food before it affects her weight. She is likewise constantly preoccupied both with the means of obtaining sufficient food to binge on and with ways of getting rid of it.

In compulsive eating, the woman usually eats excessively without being physically hungry, often in secret, gets fat and endlessly goes on and off diets, usually in the end putting on more and more weight. Compulsive eaters usually have a deep-seated fear of being thin.

Anorexics usually lose so much body weight that they stop menstruating, look like skeletons, and may even die. Bulimics do not lose quite so much weight and may look thin but normal: they usually manage to seem as if everything is all right, and binge secretly. Compulsive eaters tend to get fat and self-conscious.

An attitude to food which is defined as an eating disorder is any eating pattern where there is something going on in relation to the food other than the satisfaction of hunger, any situation where we eat or do not eat certain foods for reasons unrelated to the food itself.

Eating disorders are one of the fastest-increasing expressions of psychological difficulties, particularly among women, and they are also on the increase among men.

Food is obviously a great locus for all sorts of emotional problems: there are people who cannot eat when other people are there, who cannot eat in restaurants; people who cannot eat when they are with people who are important to them, who cannot eat with people they dislike; people who cannot eat without choking or being sick, people who forbid themselves certain foods, or who eat till they are almost comatose in order to calm feelings of anxiety.

It is clear that at the bottom of any eating disorder there is a basic issue of self-esteem, or rather lack of it. If we have any kind of compulsive relationship to food and body size then it is clear that we are not happy with ourselves just as we are, that we think there is something wrong with us, something unacceptable about us. We may try to make ourselves thinner to feel better, we may sacrifice thinness to comfort eating and put on weight. Either way we are not looking at the real reasons for our unhappiness. Some of the problem is likely to have to do with the many different messages given about women's role in society: women are generally seen as the objects of men's gaze and desire and/or as the bountiful providers for men and families. Even in this day and age we are brought up to find worth in ourselves mainly in so far as we are attractive to and ultimately marriageable by men; the images of women who are desirable to men which are promoted by the media are of very slender women, at least over the last 30 or 40 years – during which time anorexia rates have increased so enormously. As women we find that our bodies seem not to be our own but that they are required to conform to an ideal type: we may try to meet this requirement by becoming thin, overdo it and become emaciated, or we may react against this requirement by piling on the weight in defence.

Anorexia is often associated with the onset of puberty, and it has been suggested that it is an attempt to refuse to grow into a sexual woman; there is a high incidence of anorexia in women who have been sexually abused and then have a very understandable reluctance to become sexually desirable to men. Attitudes to food may also represent conflict, particularly in women, between their roles as carers and their inability to take things in for themselves: we are taught not to have overt needs.

Sometimes it seems that the attempt to take control of food represents an attempt to take control of emotional needs. The anorexic woman tries to gain control over these by controlling her physical appetite. She doesn't want to have feelings, denies that she is needy, angry or hungry and, by adopting strenuous diet and exercise rituals, tries to turn herself into someone she finds more acceptable. The bulimic woman may also use food as a way of controlling emotion: she tries to keep out hurt by bingeing, fills herself up and then cleans herself out, first secretly satisfying and then denying the need for the comforting food and the sense of fullness. Compulsive eaters try to make themselves fat for similar reasons, denying and disguising their sexuality. Getting fat for them is about protection, boundaries, containing rage, it is an expression of protest against the media image of the ideal woman, it is about a fear of being thin because of what this may mean.

Taking control over weight and shape is a way of taking control over sexuality and the opposite sex. It is also a way of taking control over parents. Food has been used as a reward or a punishment for most of us during our childhood. We have been deprived of certain foods by war or poverty or parental decision, treated with certain foods in times of affluence or holiday. Once we are old enough to exert our own influence on the food we eat, it becomes a powerful weapon. We can refuse food as a means of refusing love or control, or of keeping a smothering love at a distance. It is a way of regaining some control for ourselves in a relationship of powerlessness. Teenage anorexics tell of how they stopped eating when a new step-parent arrived, or when they felt their parents were ignoring them, or because they wanted to assert their needs above those of their demanding parents.

These issues used not to be so prominent among men. For young men the main aim used to be, and for many still is, simply to build muscle. The old bull-worker which promised to change them from seven-stone weaklings to handsome muscle-bound hunks in a few weeks has given way to the modern gym, the expensive high-protein diet and the anabolic steroids to which many are addicted. There are clearly also a number of compulsive eaters in the male population. The phenomenon of male anorexia is relatively new and it may be, in part, a reaction to sex-stereotyping in men comparable to that experienced by women who are compulsive eaters. Some men don't want to be macho and domineering, seen only as a stud, and may unconsciously develop a male body which does not conform to the current media image.

As far as treatment is concerned, the favoured orthodox approaches to anorexia, bulimia and other eating disorders tend to treat only the symptom of food control, and therefore focus on persuading the patient to change the habit. In the case of anorexia, for instance, the patient is made to rest in bed and eat huge amounts of food in order to replace lost weight. These methods are effective in making people put on weight, and therefore in averting the immediate danger of death, but their wider consequences are more problematic.

There is little point in treating just the symptoms; we have to get behind the symptoms to find out what the behaviour means. For people who need to use food like this the eating problem has often been seen as a solution to another, deeper problem: the problem of feeling unhappy and powerless. We cannot just take away their solution; we need to help people to express what is going on, to find ways of dealing with their pain and conflict other than attacking their own bodies.

Using homoeopathic remedies to help with eating disorders approaches the person on several different levels at once: the remedy seeks both to balance the low self-esteem, fears and obsessions which may have led to such extreme measures, and to restore the appetite to normal while healing whatever may have been the physical and psychological consequences of such a regime. Hospital care or some kind of close supervision may still be necessary, depending on how advanced the situation is. The family is rarely able to help with this because in many cases it is some relationship within the family which is being tested through the eating disorder.

The following remedies may prove useful adjuncts to professional therapy. The remedy pictures will very nearly show which route a person may take in the particular expression of the eating disorder but, as with other conditions, the remedy that fits the person as a whole will be the one that works best.

ANACARDIUM ORIENTALE

The fundamental lack of self-confidence inherent in the *Anacardium* picture provides the essential soil for the development of eating disorders.

The likelihood that the focus of emotional problems may become food is increased by the fact that low blood sugar and a consequent great improvement after eating are strong features of the *Anacardium* picture. This is a person who feels much better for eating and much worse when hungry, so this is likely to be a person whose eating disorder is expressed in compulsive eating and a bingeing/dieting pattern.

This kind of pattern would be entirely consistent with the remedy picture's persistent sense of the presence of two contradictory wills, a split between two parts of the personality. This remedy may be useful for people who describe themselves as eating 'in spite of' themselves.

In so far as bingeing and dieting are forms of self-punishment, this may be another way in which food disorders conform to the self-destructive patterns of the *Anacardium* personality.

ARSENICUM ALBUM

This personality type is perfectionist and overactive, and easily becomes obsessional. She likes to be active and elegant and is therefore likely to be attracted to the current slender image of the 'perfect' woman.

A desperate need to control her environment, and severe anxiety produced by feeling out of control, are the most marked characteristics of *Arsenicum*; the will to take control of emotional and bodily needs by becoming anorexic may emerge from these strong feelings.

Her obsessive perfectionism as well as her capacity for attention to detail will make it possible for this sufferer to stick to a rigid diet and exercise programme, so much so that she will be in serious danger of becoming a true anorexic.

She is naturally thin and a quick metabolizer of food, so her dieting will be successful; she will emaciate quickly.

Self-harm is also associated with the *Arsenicum* remedy picture, and with eating disorders as well: the person may cut herself with a knife or do herself some other injury.

In addition it is a feature of the *Arsenicum* remedy picture that the affected person often cannot stand the sight and smell of food, feels full no matter how little she has eaten, and has strong food sensitivities. She has a fear of suffocating on food, of being poisoned, and is in general very anxious around food – all symptoms that are very much part of the anorexic picture. Sometimes this may express itself not in open anorexia but in food allergies or sensitivities.

CALCAREA CARBONICA

The person of this type tends constitutionally to be stocky and obese; he very easily puts on a flabby sort of weight, he will say that he only has to look at food to gain the pounds. He tends to overeat and is not very physically active. He may be a person who is careless of his appearance because he undervalues himself, or who eats for comfort and piles on the weight. He may also eat to keep his vulnerable inner self from view, not minding the weight if it stops people being interested in him. His pattern is likely to be that of compulsive eating: he likes that sense of feeling full, even to the extent of feeling better when he is constipated.

The motivation to diet may come when he begins to feel more self-conscious from being overweight than from not being, and then there is a danger of bulimia if the obsessional energy always present in *Calcarea carbonica* is harnessed at this point: he may become obsessive about health, seek exercise, and become addicted to dieting.

IGNATIA AMARA

The idealism inherent in this remedy picture may show itself in the desire to look perfect: this is the kind of personality type who becomes anorexic and takes on strenuous exercise programmes in order to live up to an ideal image; she likes to look good and be attractive to the person with whom she is passionately in love.

She may overeat, because she is inclined to suffer from a nervous hunger which is not relieved by eating: the more she eats the more she wants. She tends to gain and lose weight easily, and so can become a chronic exerciser and dieter.

Her hypersensitivity to all forms of emotional disturbance may well lead her to solace herself with food, to push down feelings of disappointment, grief and abandonment.

This is also a remedy for bulimia. Bingeing and vomiting fit with her general paroxysmal and spasmodic patterns. Her nausea is relieved by eating.

NATRUM MURIATICUM

This remedy type tends to be thin despite having a good appetite. He tends to emaciate even if he is eating well.

Because of his extreme emotional privacy and reserve, this type of person may well resort to food as a means of controlling emotions he feels very deeply, but finds difficult to express: he may tend to be bulimic rather than purely anorexic, because in bulimia he can still appear to be 'normal'; no one need know what is going on inside.

On the other hand, this personality type feels wonderful when he does not eat, and this could be a powerful incentive to the anorexic way of solving problems of unhappiness.

PLATINUM METALLICUM

The *Platina* type is obviously at risk of developing an eating disorder. She tends to be thin and nervous in any case, and her compulsive, haughty superiority (covering a very low self-esteem and deep despair), her driving need for sexual contact and her desire to dress extravagantly would all lead to a demand to have the perfect figure, perfectly clothed and capable of attracting everyone.

Her constitutional tendency to have a distorted sense of size would encourage a distorted perception of her appearance.

The high possibility of there having been sexual abuse in the background of such a personality adds to the chances of developing an eating disorder.

Self-harm is characteristic of this remedy picture: she is liable to attack herself with a knife, a self-destructive act often associated with anorexia. In the remedy picture there is disturbance of the appetite – from sadness, boredom or despair – and there is also ravenous, uncontrollable eating accompanied by feelings of self-hatred and/or hatred of everyone around her.

Some of the provers (the people who experimented with the effects of taking *Platina*) ate compulsively while engaged in the experiment. One can imagine the terror of the *Platina* personality if she began to put on weight: she would be almost bound to get into a binge/purge pattern.

PULSATILLA NIGRICANS

The *Pulsatilla* personality is extremely emotional, dependent, comfort-seeking, liking the kind of food that children like and adults return to under stress for comfort: pastries, cakes, ice-cream. Such people are also subject to many obsessions and fantasies relating to food, imagining that certain items of food are not fit to be eaten by human beings.

Characteristically they eat to make themselves less depressed, then they begin to put weight on, become afraid they won't be liked, and diet to take off the weight. They are indecisive, however, and can't stick to the diet so they may have to resort to making themselves sick – and thus get caught up in the bulimic pattern.

They may become anorexic or bulimic out of their reluctance to become sexual. They are averse to and fearful of the opposite sex, even horrified by them, cannot endure the idea of marriage, so the development of eating disorders in this context may clearly be related to an unwillingness to engage sexually or in any mature relationship with others. *Pulsatilla* tends to have difficulties with puberty in any case; it is sometimes delayed and, in women, menstruation may be slow to start.

STAPHYSAGRIA

Staphysagria is characterized by suppressed indignation, resentment and pent-up anger. One of the ways this personality may suppress feelings is by eating a lot of sweets, chocolate and creamy things. Then she makes herself vomit out of guilt. Fear of gaining weight may then lead her into a bingeing and vomiting cycle.

The importance of sexual abuse in the development of the *Staphysagria* picture should sound a warning of the likelihood of the development of an eating disorder. In severe anorexia the withdrawal from food is often a form of self-punishment for obsessional sexual ideas.

SULPHUR

This remedy picture is of a person who is always hungry (except at breakfast time) and has a constant craving for food, especially sweet foods and snack foods, and alcohol. There are great swings in appetite, with a very low-energy, hungry period around 11 a.m.

Such people suffer from nausea and weakness if meals are delayed, so are likely to overeat.

Sulphur is useful for cases of bulimia, and perhaps even more so for the sort of absent-minded, alcoholic anorexia.

Chapter Eleven

GRIEF AND LOSS

Grief is not an illness but a normal reaction to loss, and it can indeed eventually prove a point of growth. It is, however, a very lonely state. It is also an extremely difficult emotion to manage, including as it might other feelings of despair, guilt, anger, terror, a sense of one's own mortality and an almost obsessional tendency to recall the lost person. Sometimes it is too difficult to grieve, and we just cut off from the whole process. We go underground and pretend we are all right; indeed, we believe that we should be. Our culture supports this. Even the well-meaning attempts to help us grieve, which talk of 'stages' and 'times of mourning', may make us feel we are doing it wrong when we find that everything happens in confusion and we don't meet these milestones. The remedies indicated below will not suppress grief, they will not make it go away; they will, however, encourage and allow the process to unfold in whatever way the individual mourner needs.

Grieving can take a long time, months and even years, depending on how important the lost person was to the identity of the survivor and how much the loss puts the survivor in touch with issues of her own mortality. Mourning is a way of coming to terms with loss. Grief may seem more severe when the death is sudden, unexpected, accidental. When the process of loss is more gradual, at the end of a long illness, for instance, it is more easily (though still painfully) integrated as a relief from suffering. Really, however, we cannot say which death will be important: we may be as profoundly affected by the death of some childhood friend or carer whom we haven't seen for a long time as by the death of a partner. For many people the loss of a beloved animal is terrible, and certainly shouldn't be under-estimated or thought surprising.

The mourning process is complex and confusing. We may feel every possible emotion: anger, indignation, despair, relief, shock, abandonment, violent self-reproach, euphoria, envy. We feel unreal, as if we weren't in the world ourselves anymore, disconnected from life. We feel, on the one hand, that nothing matters anymore and, on the other, that everything matters more than it ever did. Some people feel all these things, others only some.

In the early days of mourning it is usual for there to be a consid-erable amount of self-reproach; for what we said or didn't say before the death, for what we might have done to prevent it. Sometimes we blame others: the doctor, the homoeopath, the hospital. The early phase of mourning lasts for several weeks and may include difficulty sleeping, shakiness, loss of appetite, anxiety and fearfulness, especially when alone.

All mourning is painful because death presents us with the need to come to terms with our own mortality and with clear evidence of our lack of complete power and control over life. We are rarely the same people after an important death, and we never feel the same again about our own death or life. In finally accepting the loss of the loved person or in thinking about what has happened to her or him, we also finally accept that we are not immortal, or perhaps, even more frighteningly, that we are. The sense of the shocking insta-bility of life, which is the first feeling to follow a death, may be replaced by a more philosophical acceptance of the transience of all earthly life.

After a death for many people the thin membrane between this world and the other becomes even thinner. More people than care to tell you about it may have contact with what seems to them to be the 'spirit' of the lost person, may see him the night before or the night after the death, may hear him speak or be visited by him. Many people get presentiments of a sudden death or know when someone has died though they are not with the person. It is common to dream of the lost person. This is also something which shakes us to the root of our being.

Anniversary reactions are important too: these are unconscious psychological reactions to an earlier loss, miniature mourning reactions occurring at the time of year of the original death. These kinds of reactions happen over a number of years after the original trauma, and are marked by periods of flatness and depression, anxiety even. They may not be recognized by the person involved, who may not even be aware of the date.

Our immediate response to grief has improved in recent years. It is not very long ago that we were expected to 'get over it' in a matter of days, that children weren't allowed to go to funerals and boys were told not to cry. We are better, these days, at allowing the process to run its course. However, mourners are still often rushed: you may be allowed a few weeks now instead of a few days, but still there comes a point quite soon when people think you should have got over it, expect you to be fully functioning again, when they suggest you take some tablets if you're still not sleeping and, on the whole, avoid mentioning it.

This is counter-productive, however, because grief needs to be experienced and worked through in order to be left behind. The best thing to do is to allow the grief to be experienced but support yourself or whoever is affected with the appropriate homoeopathic remedy.

People are often reluctant to take remedies when in grief; they feel that they must work through it 'on their own'. Using homoeopathic remedies will not bypass the mourning process, it will help you to live through it more easily and deal with it more consciously. The remedies will not mask deep feelings, they will simply help you not to be completely overwhelmed by grief. They may also help you gain some control over the severe anxiety and panic which may follow in the loneliness of loss.

ACONITUM NAPELLUS

Aconite is indicated in cases of sudden death where shock and panic are uppermost. The person may be fearful of his own imminent death, and may view the world as a hostile place. A similar fear and shock reaction may recur at anniversaries if this was the dominant feature at the time of the death.

ARSENICUM ALBUM

An acute, agitated, restless state of mourning with fears of death and a sense of her own future death characterizes the *Arsenicum* grief reaction. The ultimate loss of control in death terrifies the *Arsenicum* personality, who is so needful of keeping control. She is very liable to reproach herself, to think that there was something she could have done. She is also liable to reproach others, to blame the hospital and even consider legal action. This is all part of the mourning process. She will feel very lonely and abandoned and will probably suffer from insomnia and very anxious dreams.

AURUM METALLICUM

This is indicated for people who are very severely affected by grief, full of self-reproach and hopelessness, who will not be consoled or reassured: 'What is there to live for now that the person I lived for is gone?' They will blame themselves, there will have been something they could have done better. This is the person who may kill himself impulsively after a significant bereavement.

CALCAREA CARBONICA

This is one of the best remedies for sorrow and grief. This person will tend to overidentify with the dead person, might imagine what it is like to be dead, in the grave or in the flames. She will become sleepless from imagining terrible things, might become confused, unable to collect her thoughts, unable to follow what people are saying to her. She might also become over-sensitive, easily startled and anxious as a result of her loss. She lacks the resilience to overcome an emotional shock.

IGNATIA AMARA

This is the most commonly indicated remedy in the first stages of grief: it contains all the contradictions of the grieving state in its picture: the mixture of sighs, tears and laughter, anger, anxiety, fear and extravagant expression of emotion side by side with a silent sadness which cannot be properly expressed, and which is visibly held in. You may see the mixed picture or you may see one or other of these emotions more strongly represented.

The person who needs *Ignatia* has usually completely identified with the dead or lost person and now feels that he can't exist alone. This will be a stage in any grief process, but for the person who needs *Ignatia* deeply this may be the most difficult stage to pass through. There may be a feeling of complete loss of direction, of total emptiness. There may seem to be nothing left but obsessive thinking of the beloved, an almost wilful attachment to grief as the only thing that preserves the relationship.

This kind of grief can cause menstrual periods to stop. There is much sighing, yawning and 'contradictory' behaviour: laughter and tears, anger and despair.

LACHESIS

Lachesis is an important grief remedy, when the grief has been long-lasting. You may see the passionate, dramatic side of this state in connection with grief, the Greek tragedy reaction to death and loss. This person may turn to drink in her effort to come to terms with loss. She will also have an almost clairvoyant awareness of other people's feelings, which will make her very vulnerable at times. She will be liable to get ill from grief. Her passionate nature attaches itself strongly to people, despite her fear of being betrayed: death is the ultimate betrayal and brings out anger, passion and fury as well as a collapse into despair.

NATRUM MURIATICUM

This is indicated where grief has been pervasive and long-lasting, when people have never been well since the death, or when thoughts of the dead one will not disappear. There is a strong sense of something very precious having been stolen, and such people cannot let it go from their memory. They need to be alone with their grief, it is like a deep and secret wound which they gradually learn to conceal, as they conceal all emotions. It is often needed when people have been unable to grieve at the time of the death, for whatever reason.

These sufferers develop illnesses from mourning the past; they cannot seem to recover from it for an inordinately long time. Their natural difficulty in expressing anger may be partly responsible for their inability to let go.

PHOSPHORUS

This is one of the major remedies for grief. Those affected will feel grief strongly, as they feel all emotions. The loss may also be unbearable because of their great need for people to anchor them to the world. This remedy may be particularly useful for those who are troubled by the strange phenomena that may surround a death. Hypersensitive to all external impressions, they will pick up all others' emotions too, as well as information coming through from other worlds.

PULSATILLA NIGRICANS

This is indicated where grief remains unexpressed in a normally emotionally expressive person. Loss, particularly of an important family member, is devastating for the *Pulsatilla* type, who needs constant support and reassurance. It threatens their whole defence strategy of dependence, particularly if they relied heavily on the person now dead.

SEPIA

This is one of the most deep-acting remedies. The grief will be marked by extreme fatigue, and will be worse in the evening and as the day draws on. Irritability is also marked and accompanies a flat indifference to all, especially those best loved. The emotional apathy characteristic of *Sepia* may develop in response to grief: the person may become indifferent to everyone and withdraw completely. Grief can cause periods to stop, too. Here, as with *Natrum muriaticum*, grief may turn into a deep depression which may last far beyond the normal time of mourning.

STAPHYSAGRIA

This remedy may be useful for a reserved grief where the bereaved person has difficulty experiencing or expressing the anger associated with loss. The *Staphysagria* state often comes on after the person has suffered many losses. He will react by blaming himself, feeling unworthy of the dead person.

Chapter Twelve

SLEEPLESSNESS

Sleeplessness is one of the worst of disturbances to bear; it is also very common. Vast numbers of us will suffer from it at some time in our lives and many people never feel they get a good night's sleep. For most people, however, sleeplessness is intermittent and often caused by transient worry, over-excitement or distress.

There are many things that interfere with sleep, and many practical things that can be done about it. You can make sure that your sleeping space is comfortable and heated to the right temperature, you can try to create a habit of going to bed at the same time every night so that your body clock is ready for it. You can cut caffeine out of your diet completely (this means cutting out not only coffee but also chocolate and tea). Don't work or watch stimulating television just before bed. Hot, milky drinks seem to help sleep, perhaps because of the calcium or because they prevent our blood sugar levels from falling during sleep (so we don't wake out of hunger).

Sleeping tablets undoubtedly help for a while, but they are highly addictive and also cause drowsiness and sometimes depression the following morning.

Exercise generally improves sleep over a period (exercise taken in the daytime rather than last thing at night).

There are numerous herbal remedies available which help sleep because of their mild sedative effect: valerian and passiflora are the best known and probably the most effective. They do not appear to cause the morning-after hangover that orthodox medication does, nor do they appear to be addictive.

There are many remedies with sleeplessness prominent in their picture, but as with all other conditions, insomnia is only part of a larger picture which should be looked at carefully before prescribing. The advantage of using homoeopathic remedies to help with sleep is that they will also begin to address whatever emotional or physical condition is the immediate cause of the insomnia.

In this list I have included two homoeopathic remedies (*Arnica* and *Coffea*) that do not appear elsewhere in this book because they are so well indicated for sleeplessness that it would be a pity to leave them out.

ACONITUM NAPELLUS
This is the remedy for sleeplessness following a shock, fright or panic, accompanied by restlessness, nightmares, free-floating fears or the specific fear of dying. It may be especially useful for children who cannot settle down, or for the restless insomnia often experienced in old age.

ARGENTUM NITRICUM
This is useful for sleeplessness that stems from anticipatory anxiety, such as before a holiday, a journey, or an examination.

ARNICA MONTANA
Arnica is for sleeplessness that comes of being overtired. The person is fidgety and the bed feels too hard. It may be indicated also in sleeplessness that stems from jet lag.

The person may be drowsy all day and unable to sleep at night, or may have anxious dreams and an unrefreshing sleep, waking quite agitated from these dreams (of animals, of being chased).

ARSENICUM ALBUM
This is for sleeplessness arising from general anxiety or nervousness, or mental effort. When the person first lies down to sleep she may be anxious; attacks of anxiety at night may drive her out of bed. She will be restless. She may wake between midnight and 3 a.m., restless, worried and apprehensive. Sleep can be disturbed by anxious dreams and nightmares of the dead, of danger, of pursuit, or by foreboding dreams of fire or danger. There is a danger that the

person may become suicidal from continued lack of sleep.

CALCAREA CARBONICA

This is particularly useful when children are sleepless, where there is a real fear of going to bed and to sleep because of their fear of the dark, of being alone and of their dreams. The child may have 'night terrors' and wake up screaming from the horrible faces and frightening creatures he sees in his dreams. In adults this kind of sleeplessness can be brought on by having heard upsetting news or seeing a disturbing film before bed.

COFFEA CRUDA

This is the remedy for insomnia caused by an overactive mind, when the person cannot 'switch' off for having ideas; also useful for sleeplessness that stems from excitement, happiness, or drinking too much tea or coffee.

IGNATIA AMARA

Insomnia that arises from grief, upset, disappointed love, excitement or any kind of distress is the hallmark of this remedy. The person might sigh in her sleep, or may have nightmares; he may be a very light sleeper, hearing every tiny sound.

LACHESIS

Sufferers needing this remedy can be sleepy without being able to sleep, or chronically sleepless without needing much sleep. Their insomnia arises from an overactive mind or from a fear of sleep: they may wake choking and suffocating in the night and come to fear sleep. Many symptoms in the *Lachesis* picture are worse after sleep, so there is often a reluctance to go to sleep for fear of feeling worse on waking. Also, sufferers may be reluctant to sleep because night is their most productive time.

They may be unable to get to sleep until 1 or 2 a.m., yet they often can't go back to sleep if they wake after midnight.

LYCOPODIUM CLAVATUM

This personality type has a mind that is very active at bedtime, going over and over work done during the day and worrying about it so that it is difficult to get to sleep. Once asleep he sleeps well, though he may talk and laugh in his sleep. He doesn't usually remember his dreams. He may wake at 4 a.m.

NUX VOMICA

Sleeplessness here may be the result of great mental strain, excitement, an overactive mind, irritability, anger, distressing thoughts, sensitivity to noise, too much food or alcohol, or withdrawal from alcohol or sleeping tablets. When it comes the sleep may be in fits and starts.

The key symptom is waking at around 3 or 4 a.m., lying awake thinking of all sorts of things and then falling asleep just as it is time to get up. Or the person may wake up and get out of bed for a while, do some work and then go back to bed just before it is time to get up again.

PHOSPHORUS

This is indicated for sleeplessness caused by imagination and excitement. Fears of the dark and of ghosts and a generally apprehensive state of mind may make sleep difficult or unsatisfying, with many anxious dreams; the affected person may sleepwalk.

PULSATILLA NIGRICANS

Difficulty getting to sleep in a warm or dark room, or if alone, characterizes the *Pulsatilla* insomnia. The sufferer may lie awake from worry, with one idea or problem running through her mind. Sometimes this sleeplessness can come from overeating or from rich food before bed.

The sufferer is restless in bed, waking hungry in the early hours and then falling asleep after eating.

SILICA

This sleeplessness can come on for a number of reasons: an overactive mind, after intercourse, because of a headache or strong pulsations of the body, from coldness of the feet, a rush of blood to the head, or a perceived 'hardness' of the bed.

SULPHUR

Sleeplessness here arises largely from an overactive mind, a great flow of thoughts preventing sleep. The insomniac tends to prefer to go to bed late anyway and enjoys working and reading late at night. He is drowsy during the day but wakeful at night. If he falls asleep he may wake at 3 or between 5 and 6 a.m. with a big idea, excitement or worry. When he finally gets to sleep he likes to sleep late into the morning, and then can hardly be aroused he sleeps so heavily. He feels lethargic after over-sleeping and likes cat-napping, and is better for these short sleeps.

His sleep may often be disturbed by anxious or horrific dreams which wake him with a start.

THUJA OCCIDENTALIS

This is for those who are persistently sleepless. They are restless and talk incessantly, especially by moonlight. When they sleep they may dream of dead people, or their sleep is disturbed by anxious, amorous, sometimes frightful dreams, often of falling from a height. There is a tendency to wake at about 4 a.m. and stay awake. *Thuja* is also good for sleeplessness that arises after having a vaccination.

Chapter Thirteen

ANGER, IMPATIENCE
AND VIOLENT THOUGHTS

The free expression of anger is difficult for most of us. It is named as a 'bad' or 'negative' emotion, even a sin, and we are usually trained out of it from an early age. We may allow ourselves to be snappy and irritable, but not really angry. It is probably only as very small children that we ever really had the luxury of an uncomplicated venting of anger and rage. However, in one way or another, we still have to deal with the feelings which produced the anger in the child, and how we do it can often make the difference between health and illness.

Adult feelings of anger usually arise in response to frustration of some kind, or feelings of being belittled or unappreciated. If they can be expressed, as in a safe relationship for example, and the feelings beneath the anger can be heard, then the anger will usually die away and whatever is causing the frustration may be dealt with in one way or another. Life continues. If the feelings cannot be expressed, which is more usual, then the frustration will continue to mount while the suppression of anger causes, eventually, depression or ulcers, or some other form of illness that the individual may be predisposed to acquire.

The knowledge that suppressing anger may lead to illness has led to the emergence of the therapeutic cliché that it is 'good to express anger'. However, one has to ask: 'good for whom?' The uncontained expression of anger may be briefly good, even exhilarating, for the person who expresses it, but it is rarely so good for the people on the other end of it, and its ripple effects can last a long time.

While it is undoubtedly better for an individual's emotional health to be aggressive rather than depressive, anger needs to be expressed in a context of understanding. We need to be clear that we are expressing anger appropriately, towards the person to whom it belongs. This is often impossible because the true origin of adult anger is often located in old childhood injuries. Thus our current friends and family get the anger we never expressed to parents and teachers.

Modern books and therapies have encouraged women particularly to express their anger. This has been necessary because women have traditionally been more suppressed by society in their expression of anger than men. It has become a cliché that men are allowed to express their anger more than women: they are regarded as 'standing up for themselves' if they express anger, whereas women are regarded as being 'strident' and 'irrational'.

In fact, however, anger is difficult for both sexes. Men may seem to express it more freely, but this often leads them into violence, the break-up of relationships or trouble with the law. Women, socialized into denying it, frequently get depressed instead. The danger for women is that they will over-suppress, for men that they will over-express, act out and even create physical damage through their anger. In neither case, usually, is the real issue being addressed. The expression or non-expression of anger simply replaces the issue. For both sexes it seems that it is crucially important to find a way of expressing or dealing with anger that is not destructive either of the self or others. This usually involves being aware of frustration or the beginnings of anger in ourselves and expressing it at that point, before expression becomes too dangerous.

What causes us to suppress anger is frequently the feeling we have that our anger is so great and so dammed up that if we began to express it we would destroy the whole world. We often feel just like an angry baby looks, red-faced and bursting with fury. Why? Because someone didn't shut the door quietly or was late home? Just as a baby's anger is usually about not getting a need met, that is usually what ours is about – but we can't acknowledge that anymore and have to displace it, telling ourselves that we are angry because of what the Government has done, or what the next-door neighbour said, rather than look at what we feel about what that other has done, what his or her action has made us feel and how that can be addressed. We may feel angry if we feel unseen, if we feel undervalued in some way, or if we are stopped in our forward progress in life, or if we are attacked. We may suppress this anger, masking it with hurt. We may say we are hurt when we are angry: it may be easier to cry.

Some people may have a different relationship to anger and may be able to express it: anger may be the only form of emotional expression that someone who has grown up in a violent household knows. Such people are likely, consciously or unconsciously, to look for occasions for getting angry, even for fighting. Feeling anger is probably better than feeling nothing. If they are angry they know they are alive. These people often get trapped into being able to express anger only, and are not able to reach their softer feelings, not able to say that they are hurt.

We have all met people who seem to be in a permanent state of low-level anger, continuously critical and sarcastic. Other people may be very self-righteous in anger, often appearing to think they are entitled to be so and very hard to contradict. Others get angry about the state of the world. When we meet such people we almost always ask ourselves 'Why? What is being covered up by this anger? Are they afraid to be tender, soft? Whom are they really angry with?' Expressed anger often seems to be a protection, a mask for some other, softer emotions, perhaps feelings of vulnerability and hurt in someone who does not feel that it is safe to be vulnerable.

The remedy pictures discussed below cover a wide range of ways of expressing frustration and irritability, from slight testiness to frank violence. Various remedy pictures reflect various ways of being angry, and taking the remedy may balance out the emotions enough for us to find a creative expression for them.

ANACARDIUM ORIENTALE

You may see three different modes of the expression of anger in *Anacardium*, all of which emerge in response to feelings of very low self-esteem and appalling lack of self-confidence.

One mode of anger will be fairly random aggression, wild anti-social behaviour as seen in people who like to get into fights, brawls, look for trouble. Often fighting and winning is the only way such a person can feel at all confident: violence is a defence against feeling inadequate. The keynote is an irresistible desire to curse and swear; and in mental breakdown this cursing may become completely involuntary.

The second mode is bullying behaviour. Bullies put outside themselves their own insecurity and powerlessness, and attack these 'weaknesses' in others. They have usually been hurt, attacked and bullied themselves and when they become bullies they can destroy the part of themselves that has been hurt, asserting power over themselves.

The third mode is expressed by swearing. A keynote of *Anacardium* is the irresistible desire to curse, which may emerge as the expression of a desire for revenge after humiliation.

ARSENICUM ALBUM

This remedy picture displays a cold, calculated, self-righteous anger, the critical parent personified. There will be no angry outbursts but a lot of carping, controlling criticism. This censorious attitude stems from an underlying terrifying anxiety but emerges and appears as arrogant, censorious, complaining, judging behaviour. This personality does not suffer fools gladly: she knows she is good at what she does and is quick to blame and put others in the wrong. She is full of righteous indignation.

She will normally be angry and critical in a quiet and controlled way. She often has impulses to stab and kill, though she normally inhibits them. However, she is liable to get openly angry and want to hurt and kill, especially when she feels that she or her family is threatened.

CALCAREA CARBONICA

Although the most commonly seen aspect of *Calcarea carbonica* is that of the systematic, stolid, anxious and conscientious plodder, there is an excitable, irritable side to the remedy picture too, very commonly seen in children. *Calcarea carbonica* is not usually directly aggressive but is very obstinate, and this is the state children may get into. They have constant temper tantrums, scream and shout and won't do as they are told. It can look very like the *Stramonium* symptom picture.

This remedy is also useful for hyperactive, food-sensitive children, making them much calmer.

IGNATIA AMARA

The person who needs *Ignatia* may be prone to fits of anger and can become very critical, unreasonable, irritable and angry when under emotional stress. He can become quarrelsome, selfish and impossible to please, especially when contradicted or reproached in any way. This state is usually swiftly over, spasmodic, like most *Ignatia* moods.

The sufferer can have very irritable reactions to a lot of things: to people smoking, to things going slightly wrong or out of control. He will hit the ceiling over what seems very little. He tends to cry when he is angry.

LACHESIS

The passionate nature of the *Lachesis* personality often expresses itself in an imperious irritation, accompanied by hatred and anger. There is no inhibition in the expression of these violent emotions. This personality type's anger often emerges in response to scorn, rejection or attack of any kind and she becomes maliciously, vengefully angry, even vitriolic. She is very articulate and convincing in anger.

Her anger is very likely to become uncontrollable before periods and in the menopause. If she has to control her anger for some reason she is likely to develop high blood-pressure.

LYCOPODIUM CLAVATUM

People who need *Lycopodium* frequently act in a haughty and domineering manner, even though they are inwardly unsure of themselves, full of fears and feelings of inferiority. They can be irritable and impatient, taking a sarcastic, domineering attitude to others which they barely conceal at times. They are often those who are tyrannical at home and charming away from home. They can be cruel, arrogant and egotistical. They are liable to sudden angry explosions of temper, are very quick to take offence at any imagined slight or insult, dwell on injuries (real or imagined) and harbour resentment. They will pick quarrels and will bully (usually verbally) those who can't fight back.

NUX VOMICA

The impatience of *Nux vomica* is deep-seated, habitual and permanent. It usually expresses itself in spasms of anger and irritability and is likely to emerge in response to frustration, being contradicted or impeded in any way, or to any imagined slight reprimand, criticism or insult. This type of personality can be very irascible, bossy and domineering, quite a blustering bully when in these moods. His temper can be uncontrollable, but it is usually quickly roused and quickly subsides. The violence can be verbal or can quickly erupt into a physical outburst, the person throwing and smashing things or lashing out at people.

PLATINUM METALLICUM

There is a lot of anger and irritability in the *Platina* picture. The most characteristic symptoms of the remedy are pride, haughtiness, arrogance and contempt. People who need this remedy, act in a pompous, egotistical way and are frequently rude and insulting to others, whom they regard as inferior. They are irritated by trifles and sulk over petty things. They are easily offended and can mope for a long time. They suffer from a desire to kill those close to them, those they love most. Being angry and irritable keeps them from falling into despair.

PULSATILLA NIGRICANS

The *Pulsatilla* personality has mental and physical states that are subject to frequent, quick changes – from complacent sweetness to irritable, fidgety impatience. If hurt she can get quite cross and attacking from time to time, but rarely sustains an angry mood because she quickly dissolves in tears. If she cannot get her own way by being sweet and pleasant she is inclined to become more and more selfish and demanding. She can become discontented, capricious and peevish. Her jealousy and suspicion can also rouse her to anger or, more likely, a quiet malice. She can be quick to take offence.

SEPIA

People who need *Sepia* are frequently identified by their irritability and bad temper. They can suffer outbursts of anger and hatred,

wanting to scream. Primary causes are overwork and exhaustio
being drained. They can go either into indifference, apathy an
collapse or into irritability and quarrelsomeness. They are inclined to
be vehement, can be spiteful and extremely intolerant of contradiction, get nasty or fly into a passion of self-justification.

STAPHYSAGRIA

This kind of person seems so nice and yet you feel he might be
capable of great rage and real nastiness. He will normally appear to
be very pleasant and unassuming: this is a cover for a deep resentment which you may sometimes sense, though it is not clearly
expressed. Occasionally, there may be an outburst of uncontrollable
anger and indignation, long suppressed. Then this normally quiet
and compliant person may throw things.

Suppressed anger and resentment may strike deeper and manifest
as depression, even suicidal depression with deep feelings of worthlessness.

STRAMONIUM

The chief characteristic of the *Stramonium* picture is the intensity of
its anger and violence: it will emerge in a rush and be impossible to
restrain. The violence is verbal, with constant compulsive cursing
and swearing. It is also active: the person may smash things, tear
clothes, destroy whatever is around to destroy. It will come on
suddenly and settle down just as suddenly when the energy has been
expended, but it is marked by being totally out of control and
cannot be reasoned with or restrained except by force while it is
going on.

SULPHUR

At its worst the *Sulphur* state's self-absorption makes this person
easily offended – if challenged she responds with irritation and
criticism. She enjoys intellectual argument and will argue about anything, sometimes becoming quite quarrelsome, just for argument's
sake. She relates to other people by arguing and discussing things
with them, and enjoys getting people worked up, often not noticing
that she is causing them distress. At the same time she dislikes people who offend her and can become quite morose and suspicious.

This person has an excitable, volcanic nature and can be quick to anger and to penitence. She may display sudden eruptions of temper which subside quickly. She gets impatient with those she sees as slower-minded.

Chapter Fourteen

BREAKDOWN OR BREAKTHROUGH

The pages of a self-help book are not perhaps where you would expect to find advice on the treatment of the conditions called mania and schizophrenia. Such serious emotional crises in the lives of individuals should, of course, be treated by professionals and over the long term, not as a matter of first-aid.

However, it seems to be increasingly common for people to suffer such episodes, and since conventional treatment has little to offer apart from physical protection and drugs, the families and friends of those suffering are often left without help. This chapter will give some indication of how to recognize some of these 'psychotic' states and respond to them with the appropriate remedies, hopefully before the state has become too overwhelming and therefore leaving little alternative to heavy medication. It will also give some indication of the long-term possibilities of using homoeopathy in the treatment of severe mental breakdown.

Psychotic breakdown takes place when people are mentally disturbed to the extent that they cannot control the eruption of the contents of their unconscious – in other words they cannot control their thoughts and behaviour. Characteristically this state is signalled by disordered thoughts, hallucinations of various kinds, seeing visions, smelling smells, hearing voices, having delusions as to one's own strength and importance, and experiencing feelings of persecution. The state may first make itself known when the sufferer becomes very withdrawn, more and more isolated from other people, mistrusting others and finding it difficult to relate to them –

perhaps even becoming silent and motionless, eventually catatonic. Whatever form it takes the person substantially loses contact with ordinary reality; he is not living in the same reality as the rest of us. In these states people may be diagnosed as suffering from mania or schizophrenia of various kinds.

Manic depression (or bipolar disorder as it is properly called) seems to be an exaggerated version of the mood swings with which many of us are familiar as features of everyday life. Ordinarily they are caused by the weather, hormonal disturbance, food sensitivities, various disappointments and triumphs or by unknown agents. Sometimes they just come and go of their own accord. As children we get away with them if we are lucky; as adolescents they are taken to be characteristic of that trying time. In adults they are regarded as unacceptable. You have to be very individualistic or eccentric to get away with having severe mood swings as an adult.

In ordinarily moody people, optimism is followed by pessimism and depression, with a rapid alternation between high and low moods, or there may be a more settled low, depressed state which is interrupted from time to time by an elated, excitable hyperactivity and creativity which makes all the lowness seem (temporarily) worthwhile. At some point this pattern may attract the label manic-depression, or bipolar disorder. If it is not controlled in some way the depressions may become more and more marked, deeper and darker, while the periods of elation may become positively danger-ous: the hyperactivity and creativity being applied to completely unrealizable aims, with excessive talking and laughter, overspending, and delusions of grandeur or even of persecution which resemble those of schizophrenia. The person's career or family life may be adversely affected by his excessive actions.

Even though mania may be extremely destructive, its creative potential can make some people idealize it. It is very hard to roman-ticize schizophrenia, however, though there was a long period in the 1960s when this was done. In what is called schizophrenia the person concerned is overwhelmed by the unconscious, he cannot do anything except drown. His identity or selfhood shatters; he is unable to distinguish between inner feelings and thoughts and outer reality.

In schizophrenia the parts of our personality which we all have, such as our unkind part or our religious part, are reified, seen as other beings and placed outside ourselves, projected, experienced as alien to us rather than part of us. While we are healthy neurotics we may *imagine* that people are looking at us in the street; when we fall over the edge into psychosis we *know* they are looking at us and, what is more, that they are plotting to kill us. What we do is split off the part of ourselves that feels self-destructive and project it outwards, creating an outside personality so that we can feel persecuted from outside of ourselves rather than from within. The feelings of persecution may stay at this level (of feelings and delusion) or, in very rare cases (which inevitably make the new spaper headlines) they may become so extreme that a person will get a gun and go out and kill the people who are 'out to get him'. More usually we turn our hostility against ourselves.

While we are suffering from such feelings we are bewildered, depressed, withdrawn, feel dead and empty inside and emotionally flat, seeing no meaning in anything. We are subject to delusions and hallucinations in a terrifying world in which our thoughts become our reality.

Little is known for certain about why some people break down in this dramatic way, totally losing contact with reality and becoming completely overwhelmed by the breakthrough of material from the unconscious, while others, however unhappy they are and however much stress they have, stay largely in contact with everyday reality. There are many theories but these tend to change with every generation and are not reliable, particularly as they are subject to a lot of social prejudice.

However, although we don't know the fundamental cause of psychotic breakdown or what causes the predisposition to it, we do know that it may sometimes have as its immediate cause, its trigger, such things as the use of drugs (especially LSD or amphetamines, and probably Ecstasy; glue-sniffing is another, increasingly common, cause). Temporary and permanent states can be induced by alcohol abuse. Also it can happen as a result of a severe reaction to a traumatic event: shock, accident, war, acute physical trauma, loss of a job or relationship. It can as well be a feature of post-traumatic stress disorder of any origin.

A breakdown may also be seen as a form of psychospiritual crisis:

some people seem to have to go into the depths of their own unconscious in order to rearrange it for themselves and come out the other side. Carl Jung, Sigmund Freud and Wolfgang Pauli are just a few of the distinguished thinkers who have passed through a period of apparent mental breakdown as part of their personal development and been enriched by it. They were privileged to have been allowed to do so in peace. For most people, and for their friends and families, psychotic breakdown is a terrifying experience yielding very little meaning. People who are able to express themselves in an artistic way may reach its meaning through their art: Van Gogh, for instance. There are many examples of the creativity inherent in madness. However, most people can only survive it with their personality intact through the dedicated help of friends and concerned physicians: fortunately there are some of these around and many people do survive with the help of drugs in a far more comfortable way than they would once have done without them.

However, the relative success of drugs in controlling the grosser symptoms of these illnesses may be the enemy of a better outcome which might be achieved by other methods. The current labelling of such illnesses as diseases with physical causes leads to depression and frustration because it suggests that these actions originate in chemical imbalances for which there is no cure, and that symptoms can only be controlled with powerful drugs with damaging side-effects. We cannot know whether, with other help, the individual could have emerged from the other side of the crisis without need of drugs.

Treatment of people in psychotic states is, however, extremely problematic in our society. Even with the best will in the world and the best facilities, all we really know how to do is to use physical restraint in the early stages to protect the person and his family if that is needed, and then to use drugs to sedate and control the behaviour (that is, to suppress the symptoms). We have neither the time, resources nor knowledge to do anything better. Many people resume a reasonably settled and productive life after treatment, but we see on the streets of all our major cities those for whom an answer has not been found, we see them among those who beg and who sleep in doorways, giving the lie to our politicians' claims to have established a fair, just and civilized society. We cannot ignore them or imagine that any kind of humane solution has been found for whatever diagnosis we give to their condition.

There are many hints in homoeopathic remedy pictures for remedies that would help in these conditions. I include them here so that this may become common knowledge and the basis for further thought and practice, rather than out of any facile claim that homoeopathy can treat with a few tablets conditions which have tested the skills of physicians for hundreds of years. It would not be wise to attempt long-term treatment of a severely ill friend or family member without the help of a professional homoeopath.

In many ways the delusions and hallucinations that are present in remedy pictures are little clue to the particular remedy needed in a psychotic breakdown. There is such common ground between various forms of delusions and hallucinations that these symptoms, however flamboyantly expressed, do not help us to make distinctions between remedies when we are trying to prescribe. It is common in psychotic breakdown to feel double, to feel separated from the self, to hear voices, to have lascivious thoughts or delusions of persecution, to feel under threat of death, to lose hope of salvation, to believe you are someone very important or to have hallucinations of devils and Satan. When the collective unconscious overwhelms us, it does so with little respect for our individuality.

The following remedy pictures all include such bizarre symptoms; these are the pictures of some of the personality types which have the potential for this kind of breakdown. These are likely to be the most effective acute remedies, but differentiation between them will usually need to be made on other, more constant general and characteristic symptoms of both the remedy and the person.

ANACARDIUM ORIENTALE

For an *Anacardium* personality in mental breakdown, the ever-present sense of a split between two contradictory wills, two parts of the personality – the tormented conflict between good and evil, angel and devil – is reified. Voices are sometimes heard from outside, telling the sufferer to kill in the name of god. There is a marked paranoia with delusions of persecution and intrusive thoughts. The person may have hallucinations that demons, spirits and monsters are attacking her, that Satan must be destroyed; or she may have delusions that one of her family is possessed by the devil.

She suffers from dramatic alternations of mood: deep guilt and torment about her soul and salvation alternating with mania, maliciousness and impulsiveness.

What is *characteristic* of the *Anacardium* way of being with these symptoms is their wild violence. The person may curse and swear compulsively and be unrestrainedly angry and violent. She has lost the sense of reality which normally controls her behaviour. There is a danger of suicide brought on by a desperate desire to get rid of the intrusive thoughts.

ARSENICUM ALBUM

This remedy contains within itself the pattern of bi-polar disorder, with its restless, enthusiastic, driven activity followed by exhaustion. Sufferers are always in a hurry and restless, swing easily between fear/anxiety and excitement/irritability, and have lots of ideas over-flowing from their brain.

The *Arsenicum* remedy picture also contains the pattern of the illness labelled as paranoid schizophrenia: the tendency to suspect that friends have been offended and hate one. There may come a time when this acquires the status of a delusion, when sufferers may become convinced that they are being watched, pursued by enemies, conspired against, that murder is being plotted against them and that they have to murder someone. Their normal fastidiousness and anxiety about germs and contamination may develop into the fixed idea that they are being poisoned, that rats and other vermin are all over the bed, all over the house; tormenting thoughts of disease may intrude and crowd around each other; the impulsiveness around knives may become a real desire to kill.

Whatever the disease label, you will always see beneath the symptoms the perfectionism, restlessness, meticulousness and the need for control characteristic of *Arsenicum*.

LACHESIS

In this remedy picture there is usually a restless, nervous excitement with a tendency to jealousy and suspicion. In mental breakdown you may see a severely agitated, manic state with a tendency to mock others. Sufferers are endlessly loquacious and don't stop until they have exhausted themselves and everyone else; they change the subject rapidly, have abundant ideas and flights of fancy, and are excitable and exhilarated.

You may also see an exaggeration of their natural suspiciousness into paranoia and fantasies or delusions of persecution: in general the person feels controlled and influenced by others, has delusions that he is being poisoned, that there are conspiracies against him. He thinks that he is under a powerful influence, that he will be injured, is pursued, has persistent thoughts of evil.

As his sense of identity disintegrates he begins to think he is someone else, or that he is two people.

There will always be a strong sexual component in the madness of *Lachesis*. What is characteristic is excitability in combination with suspicion, jealousy and high sexuality.

PHOSPHORUS

The kind of mental breakdown which might be associated with a *Phosphorus* state is likely to be much more peaceful (from the outside) than most. The persistent problem with establishing boundaries between oneself and others, between oneself and other worlds, will be magnified: the sufferer will see ghosts, have hallucinations of the dead, see faces, devils and other frightful images; she will hear voices, become even more clairvoyant or clairaudient than usual, and may have erotic delusions.

This remedy may also be useful in mania, where the manic behaviour is liable to take the form of doing things for other people, for example collecting vast sums of money for charity, then spending it on a holiday.

Characteristic will be the insubstantial, unearthed quality of the state, and the sufferer's strong desire for company.

PLATINUM METALLICUM

This mental state is often profoundly disturbed, with severe confusion. The characteristic tendency to look down on others and to feel elevated and proud will be exaggerated. Sufferers are very often extremely irritable and at times violent. In a manic phase they are full of their own self-importance; in the down phase they are deeply depressed. When the psychotic state is severe their body image becomes fragmented, they feel that their arm or limbs are not attached to them.

The feelings of being more important than others may overwhelm them either temporarily or permanently: they can become trapped in the condition labelled schizophrenia, feeling or having delusions that they are royalty, Napoleon, descendants of the Russian Royal family. They may have fantasies that everything is small, everybody is mentally and physically inferior, that they themselves are large and superior – they may even sense themselves growing bigger. They may develop mania.

The characteristic feature of the *Platina* breakdown, however, would be the attitude of haughtiness, combined with an obsession with sexual matters.

STRAMONIUM

This will probably be the most useful remedy to use in an acute case, at the point where there is real, undeniable breakdown, where the person goes into a highly agitated, active, driven violent state, with hallucinations, convulsions and constant uncoordinated movements. There will be restlessness, rage and a great deal of destruction and violence in this kind of psychotic state. The person will want to take off his clothes, smash things, fight, bite, tear up clothes; he will be incoherently talkative, compulsively shouting and swearing. Or, he may be silent, withdrawn and catatonic: collapsed in a heap on the floor picking at his clothes. This is the most valuable acute remedy for breakdown.

You may be able to see the picture emerging before the actual breakdown and avert it. Wherever you see glimpses of this uncontrolled eruption of deep unconscious fears with rage and violence, think of *Stramonium*. You may see the characteristic fears and anxieties of this remedy developing: fear of the dark, of cemeteries, tunnels, closed places, dogs, and/or large bodies of water.

The acute stage of *Stramonium* may resemble the picture of *Belladonna*. A *Stramonium* state may be brought on, in a susceptible person, by a frightening situation: an operation, a violent rape or attack, a bad trip on LSD or Ecstasy. Possibly even by strobe lights, because of the fear of and effect of flashing lights.

PART THREE

Materia Medica

Aconite *Aconitum napellus*
Anacardium *Anacardium orientale*
Argentum nitricum *Argentum nitricum*
Arsenicum *Arsenicum album*
Aurum *Aurum metallicum*
Calc carb *Calcarea carbonica*
Gelsemium *Gelsemium sempervirens*
Ignatia *Ignatia amara*
Lachesis *Lachesis*
Lycopodium *Lycopodium clavatum*
Natrum mur *Natrum muriaticum*
Nux vomica *Nux vomica*
Phosphorus *Phosphorus*
Platina *Platinum metallicum*
Pulsatilla *Pulsatilla nigricans*
Sepia *Sepia*
Silica *Silica*
Staphysagria *Staphysagria*
Stramonium *Stramonium*
Sulphur *Sulphur*
Thuja *Thuja occidentalis*

ACONITUM NAPELLUS

(Monk's Hood, Wolf's Bane)

EMOTIONAL AND PSYCHOLOGICAL CHARACTERISTICS
Aconite grows high up in the mountains and is extremely poisonous.
It is swept by storms, indeed its action has been likened to that of a
great storm: it comes up suddenly, sweeps over and passes away.

The symptom picture of *Aconite* is usually easy to spot in its acute
state: very fast breathing (hyperventilation), palpitations and a
flushed face, even fainting, with obvious panic, anxiety and fear.

Usually the symptoms come on suddenly, almost out of nowhere.
A person may wake up in the middle of the night from a frightening dream feeling panicky, or have a sudden attack of anxiety while
walking down the street. There is often a strong sense that a heart
attack is imminent, and a fear of immediate death: in fact, the
physical symptoms can resemble those of a heart attack so closely
that people have been taken to hospital in this state.

Aconite is the first remedy to consider in the case of severe
anxiety, panic attacks or fear, and for the after-effects of these states.
It is also a very important remedy for shock and the effects of shock,
even years later – the shock, perhaps, of having seen or been
involved in a bad accident, or of sudden bereavement, or the often
unacknowledged shock to the baby of a difficult or sudden birth. It
is never too late to give *Aconite*; even years after the event it will
begin to realign the disturbed vital force.

When we come to look at the characteristic chronic symptom
picture of *Aconite*, fear remains the dominant feature, constantly
expressed in a variety of ways. Sufferers may fear the dark, ghosts,

crowds, crossing the road or even going out on the street. They may fear intangible things: 'I don't know what'. When asleep they have nightmares and often wake up afraid. Fear of death, either immediately or at a very particular future time, is most marked.

Impatience is another noticeable feature: there is no tolerance of pain, noise, or any disturbance. The sufferer easily gets beside himself, anguished, even raving. There is great excitement accompanied by anxiety, restlessness and fear.

General and Characteristic Physical Symptoms

- Symptoms come on suddenly, violently and intensely: this may apply to complaints such as palpitations, joint pains, urinary infections, earache and all others including severe bleeding.
- Burning, tingling, shooting, 'unbearable' pains.
- Intense neuralgic pain, especially in the face (trigeminal area).
- Sudden inflammation. The picture is often seen in acute feverish illnesses, but the remedy is also effective where there are no fever symptoms. In fever the face is red, dry and flushed and the skin burning, usually without perspiration, sweat relieves. High temperatures are preceded by chill. There may be an intense thirst for large quantities of cold water. *Aconite* is well indicated in the earliest stages of almost any acute illness: colds, croup, pneumonia or any infection.

States and conditions are improved by: open air, sleep, profuse sweats.

States and conditions are made worse by: extremes of temperature, night (especially midnight).

States and conditions may be caused by: chills, exposure to cold, dry air, fear, shock.

ANACARDIUM ORIENTALE

(Semecarpus anacardium, the Marking Nut Tree)

EMOTIONAL AND PSYCHOLOGICAL CHARACTERISTICS
This remedy is made from the black corrosive juice which lies
between the shell and the kernel of the marking nut; the kernel itself
is shiny and sweet. This is a good image for the remedy, because what
we find in *Anacardium* is a strong sense of separation between the
outer appearance and the inner self. Corrosiveness is what separates
the two, the well-known vindictiveness and malice of *Anacardium*
covering the sweetness and meekness of the inner kernel.

The sense of a split in the personality is present in many remedies –
as it is present, to some degree, in many people – but it is perhaps
more rigid in *Anacardium* than in some other pictures. Most
people are vaguely aware of having various aspects of their personalities more or less hidden: in *Anacardium* one side or part is often
almost completely excluded even to the point of surprising the
person when it emerges: 'I feel like two different people,' sufferers say.

This may be perceived as a split between 'good' and 'evil,'
between the parts that are acceptable to others and those that are
not. A person may behave well, may appear to be a good person, but
may have a seriously repressed 'wicked' side. The *persona*, or social
self, is so important and what is underneath so threatening to the
personality, that even the person herself cannot admit the 'shadow'.
She cannot admit that although she is usually kind she may sometimes feel angry and cruel, so the angry and cruel part has to be
completely blocked off – emerging all the more savagely for being
blocked. Or the person may be tough and aggressive, unable to

admit, even to herself, her soft, sentimental side. A situation of moral conflict arises where there is an impulse to act cruelly and violently opposed by a conscious determination to do the right thing, or *vice versa*.

Anacardium can be a very good remedy for children with severe behavioural problems, children who get into a lot of fights, especially children who are good at home and out of control at school or *vice versa*. Adolescence is also a time when this duality is expressed in various ways, and you may also see the emergence of a suppressed side of someone while she is under the influence of drugs or alcohol. Wherever there is impulsive behaviour which seems to contradict the person's normal mode of being, there may be an indication for *Anacardium*. The person may feel herself to be under the influence of two contradictory wills. The keynote symptom of *Anacardium* exactly describes this situation – the sense that there is an angel on one shoulder, a devil on the other.

It is a useful remedy for the point in most people's lives when this shadow side begins to emerge, where the parts of ourselves which we, or others, have labelled 'bad' and suppressed begin to demand attention and integration. There is always a sense of the person having been made to be one way at the expense of the expression of another side of herself, which keeps leaking out in different ways. This may have arisen through domination at home or at school or in some other context.

Lack of self-confidence is a strong symptom. The person who needs *Anacardium* is very unsure and indecisive; she feels she cannot do anything or that she does everything wrong. She can feel completely worthless.

Weak memory is also highly characteristic, along with a dulled ability to understand. It is a useful remedy for alleviating exam panic, that mental blankness before exams when lack of self-confidence and poor memory can no longer be disguised. It can also be helpful for the effects of too much study or intellectual work. In this case the person's lack of concentration may be more general; she may always seem to be in a dream, may even feel herself to be in a dream. This kind of dreamy relationship with the mind may also come about as the result of drug use. Loss of memory for recent events is characteristic.

There is lot of *anxiety with fear*: fear of failure, fear about the future, fear of being pursued. The sufferer has fear of her own actions, of what she might do, that something dreadful will happen; she fears going insane, and may feel that someone has done something to her mind. She may feel quite suicidal from anxiety and intrusive thoughts, with an urge to shoot herself to put a stop to the internal torment and the fear of insanity.

Anacardium may also be useful when there is a more severe disturbance of the personality. It is then that the fundamental lack of self-confidence may give birth to suspicion and mistrust, to fears that people are out to get one, even to true paranoia with delusions of persecution: so-called schizophrenic states may not be far away.

In extreme cases the sense of duality may express itself in the hearing of voices, of commands to do whatever it is that has so far been suppressed: for example, this person may be convinced that 'God has told her' to go and kill or torture someone. She splits off the part of herself she finds unacceptable and projects it out into the world, and then may attempt to destroy it. She decides that it is not she who is bad, but that badness is out there, or in some member of her family.

The sufferer may develop feelings that her body does other things than the mind orders: 'It wasn't me, it was someone else inside me.' She may write one thing when meaning to write another, or do the opposite of what she intended; she may be convinced she has committed a crime, and even confess to it.

All sorts of feelings or delusions of being split in two may come up: she may have the sensation that her mind and body are separate, that she is two people. She may have the experience of leaving her body in sleep and of watching herself from the ceiling.

There is also a manic or manic-depressive application to this remedy. There are dramatic alternations of mood: deep guilt and torment about the fate of the soul and salvation, alternating with mania. During manic episodes sufferers are always wild and extravagant, compulsively cursing and swearing.

Sleep is difficult: drowsy by day, at night sleep is disturbed by vivid dreams – of fire, dead bodies, steep places and so on, so that the person wakes unrefreshed.

General and Characteristic Physical Symptoms

- The sensation of a plug or blunt object runs through all the symptoms: sensation of pressure as if by a plug (anywhere), of being stopped up (often expressed in headaches or in constipation with ineffectual urging).
- Sensations that part of the body feels cooped-up or constricted, feelings as if the legs or head were bandaged.
- Digestive system disorders: constipation, nervous dyspepsia, low blood sugar: sufferers are much better for eating and worse for missing meals. There may be an unpleasant taste in the mouth; constant thirst.
- Skin eruptions which can look like poison ivy rash; eczema from psychological causes.

States and conditions are improved by: rest, eating. The sufferer will also feel better in the evening than during the day.

States and conditions are made worse by: cold and cold draughts, exertion, an empty stomach, mental effort, hot applications, the morning hours.

States and conditions may be caused by: oppressive childhood or other relationship, excess intellectual work or sexual activity, an imminent examination, Alzheimer's disease, drugs – especially LSD.

ARGENTUM NITRICUM

(Silver nitrate)

EMOTIONAL AND PSYCHOLOGICAL CHARACTERISTICS
This remedy picture reveals a personality which is impulsive,
instinctively expressive of emotions, extravert and sociable, excitable
– the type of person who is bubbling with happiness one minute,
breaking into tears the next, who has sudden tempers and then fits
of remorse. He is sympathetic and suggestible, with a lot of vitality
and a strongly emotional nature. He gets easily flustered and very
anxious, feels hot and bothered, rushed, and 'all over the place'; he
is always in a hurry, restless, even driven. He has a strong need to
express himself and does not like to be held in – if he *is* held in he
feels trapped. He sometimes gets the feeling he is like fizzy water
trapped in a bottle – a very good way to picture this personality.

This sense of feeling trapped pervades the remedy picture: it is the
root of all its characteristic anxieties. People who need *Argentum*
get anxious in any situation which resembles a trap: crowds, closed
spaces, the middle of the row at the cinema, bridges or tunnels,
heights, tall buildings, airplanes, underground railways – anywhere
that getting out quickly would be difficult.

They need to be able to move; they are hurried and restless,
walking faster and faster for no reason. They have impulses to escape
from their trap, to jump from windows and high places, especially
over water: from cliffs or bridges. When something is arranged
for the future, again they have a sense of being trapped, limited.
They cannot bear suspense or uncertainty; they have to be able to
act, do something: waiting and anticipating is intolerable,

even when what is anticipated is pleasurable.

They particularly feel trapped and anxious in anticipation of performances or exams, and may tremble with nervous excitement, sweat, get diarrhoea. This is caused by excitability as much as fear. They worry about being late for trains or appointments. Theirs is a great sense of agitation and turbulence: they are openly fearful, apprehensive, anticipate ordeals, fear that something may happen, have fears about being alone and about their health. They are always expecting something unpleasant to happen, always wondering, 'What if...?'

Underlying this are their chronic fears of failure and of criticism, their constant doubt of their ability to succeed at anything. When they are under prolonged stress they may become mentally confused and forget things easily; they will be inclined to palpitations and trembling. This state might be chronic and constitutional, or it might be brought on temporarily by overwork, stress, studying for exams. It can also be brought on by some degenerative diseases. The sufferer's memory may start failing, he becomes prey to whatever peculiar ideas come to mind, can't get rid of them.

These fears can become obsessive and debilitating, the affected person coming to suffer from fear of his own thoughts, to be tormented by his strong imaginings. He gets panic attacks, even severe ones, and is convinced things are going to go wrong, that everything will fail, gradually becoming obsessed with this idea. He may become obsessively fearful, afraid of the panic attacks he is going to have, afraid he is going to have diarrhoea. He may become obsessed with the idea that death is imminent. He may also have anxious and foreboding dreams, and suffer from insomnia.

The sufferer may start to behave obsessively: walking only on certain stones or by certain routes, avoiding walking under ladders, fearing certain dates, or developing a lot of superstitious behaviours.

General and Characteristic Physical Symptoms

- Warm-bloodedness. Complete inability to bear heat of any kind. Sufferers feel claustrophobic in warm stuffy rooms and are better for fresh air. They are prone to sudden, profuse nervous sweats.
- Sensations that certain parts of the body feel too big, or splinter-

like sensations. These pains are sharp, come and go slowly and are often felt down the left-hand side of the body.

- Ulceration of tissues is a strong feature: there may be ulceration of the eyes, conjunctivitis, gastric ulcers with indigestion, flatulence, wind, ulcerative colitis.
- Nervous diarrhoea; Irritable Bowel Syndrome.
- A craving for salt, sugar, sweets and ice cream, all of which can cause sickness and diarrhoea. Sufferers may feel great thirst.
- Throat complaints and hoarseness are common.
- Extreme tiredness: exhaustion and trembling often come on after overwork, as do palpitations and pulsating sensations.
- Difficulties with coordination, both mental and physical. The nervous system may be badly affected: neurological conditions may be involved (especially MS).

States and conditions are improved by: cold, cold applications, company, fresh air.

States and conditions are made worse by: night, warmth and heat; they can be bad just before the menstruation period, and on waking.

States and conditions may be caused by: mental exertion, emotional stress.

ARSENICUM ALBUM

(White oxide of arsenic)

EMOTIONAL AND PSYCHOLOGICAL CHARACTERISTICS

This remedy is made from the well-known poison arsenic, used by many murderers to dispose of unwanted enemies. Small doses of arsenic are not poisonous and used to be given to horses to make their coats sleek and glossy, while women of fashion used to take it to make themselves look attractively pale. The *Arsenicum* personality may well be described as someone with a fashionable appearance, sleek, glossy hair and – at her worst – a poisoner's disposition. She is characteristically elegant, unassuming and efficient, but has a deep need to control her environment: loss of control can lead to murderous feelings.

In health the person who will eventually need *Arsenicum* is basically a perfectionist, a hard worker, organized, careful, self-disciplined, conscientious and totally reliable, whose only fault is that she expects you to be as conscientious and attentive to detail as she is. She can seem very relaxed and pleasant as long as her surroundings are in the kind of order she likes, as long as the routine she needs is established. It is important for her to know exactly what is happening, to be in control, and as long as this is achieved everyone benefits. If not, then the person can become critical and demanding, or agitated and panicky.

The need to keep meticulous control over her environment gives rise to all sorts of anxieties, centred particularly on time, health and the possibility of germs and contamination. This personality type absolutely hates unpunctuality and is always early for appointments.

She even has nightmares about arriving late, about not being ready for a journey, about missing trains or planes: these supplement her conscious, waking anxieties. She worries constantly about health – her own and that of her family – particularly about heart disease, cancer, AIDS, about whatever disease is in the public eye. She also worries about death, the future, being alone, money – almost anything which might affect her ability to stay in control of her life. The most characteristic thing about her worry is that it is completely impossible to reassure her. She is meticulously orderly and conscious of the importance of cleanliness, washes all food before she eats it and is, for instance, fastidious about the presence of pets in the kitchen.

This person is always operating at a persistent low level of anxiety and worry which she is often not aware of in herself because she tends to conceal anxiety (even from herself) by working ever harder to keep things in order. In order to survive she feels that she has to get everything right and do more all the time. She is the classic workaholic who may have a compulsive need to overwork until she drives herself into the ground, to keep going until her health breaks down. She is restless, but this restlessness is more than physical: it derives from an inner anxiety which keeps her always on the go. She finds it impossible to relax.

If her health begins to break down seriously then she may start to arrive hours early for appointments, or to worry inordinately about catching trains. Her carefulness about fitness may become an excessive concern about minor deviations in health, or even severe hypochondria: she may begin to imagine that she has every disease she reads about, moving from therapy to therapy to get support and cure, convinced that she is incurable; she may develop an agonizing fear of death, particularly from cancer. Her natural fastidiousness and orderliness may become a fanatical compulsive rigidity, a desperate attempt to keep the disorder of the external world at bay, to control an environment increasingly seen as hostile. She may become quite obsessional, tidying and cleaning for the sake of it; her sensible attention to cleanliness and hygiene may turn into an obsessional fear of germs and dirt, just as her liking for accuracy and attention to detail may become a dogmatic pedantry.

She often appears to be very selfish and indeed, behaves selfishly:

her own survival needs unconsciously making her put her own (or her family's) needs above those of all others, and fight on continually in pursuit of them. She insists on getting her needs met, on having things how she wants them; she has little tolerance of others with different needs. Within her nature there is a definite competitive element, a determined, planned pursuit of goals. She has a profound need to be self-sufficient, and a deep desire to have everything under control. Underlying all this may be a desperate fear of abandonment. She also fears poverty enormously, which can make her seem miserly and greedy.

It seems that she suppresses or represses a good deal of anger: the symptoms emerging from the unconscious reveal this. She suffers from fear of her own impulses, of harming herself or others. She may develop a fear of knives and can't have them lying around.

She is considerably agitated and restless, suffering from agoraphobia, claustrophobia and other phobias of all kinds. She fears impending evil and robbers. She has anxious dreams and nightmares: of the dead, of danger, of pursuit. She suffers from fear of the dark, of dying, of serious illness.

She is prone to panic attacks, especially if people she relies on are going away. She does not like to be alone. In acute anxiety the physical symptoms associated with *Arsenicum* are very apparent: breathlessness, restlessness, hurry, palpitations. All her anxieties and fears are worse as evening draws on, worse at night (especially between midnight and 3 a.m.), and worse when she is alone. She feels much better in company, and when occupied doing something. She may become sleepless with anxiety, not getting to sleep for reviewing the day gone by, or waking with anxious thoughts about the day to come and being unable to go back to sleep.

She can tire herself out with anxiety and overwork, working till she comes to a sort of paralysed standstill, till she is prostrate. The prostration seems out of all proportion to whatever illness it is connected with. Prostration alternates with frenetic overwork, depression with excitement.

As her health gets worse so all these symptoms become exaggerated. She becomes more and more suspicious, more and more convinced that people are out to get her. Her fears of being poisoned grow rapidly more persistent. She starts becoming genuinely paranoid and does not want people around her; she becomes hostile. There may also be exhaustion, despair of recovery and a loathing for life which may drive her to suicide.

General and Characteristic Physical Symptoms

- Restlessness, having to move about.
- Exhaustion from minor causes.
- Symptoms are mainly felt down the right-hand side of the body.
- Chilly, but uncomfortable in stuffy rooms.
- Extreme sensitivity to cold.
- Burning pains, better for heat.
- Digestive problems: sickness and diarrhoea, indigestion and heartburn, gastroenteritis.
- Sufferers are thirsty for sips of cold water, but also desire hot drinks; they crave oils, fats, sour foods.
- Thin watery (often burning) discharges.
- Ulcerative conditions (especially in the stomach and bowels) are common.
- Breathing difficulties are common (*Arsenicum* is a very important asthma remedy).
- Heart problems are common, as is high blood-pressure.
- Dry scaly skin, eczema.

States and conditions are improved by: company, heat of any kind (except in the case of headaches, which are better for fresh air), changing position.

States and conditions are made worse by: being alone, night (particularly midnight–3 a.m.), cold, cold food, iced drinks.

States and conditions may be caused by: asthma, terminal or serious illness, food poisoning, abandonment.

AURUM METALLICUM

(Gold)

EMOTIONAL AND PSYCHOLOGICAL CHARACTERISTICS
Gold is the symbol of love, hope and power, of royalty. It is the most
precious of metals. In some respects this reflects the character of
people needing *Aurum*. They experience themselves almost as
having once been royal but having fallen from a great height. Not
that they feel they are royal in the sense of being separate from and
above others, but royal in the medieval sense of having responsibilities and caring for other people.

Conscientiousness is a key characteristic of the *Aurum* personality. They tend to be over-responsible, over-conscientious,
meticulous, hardworking. They tend to devote themselves whole-
heartedly to whatever they are doing. Responsibility weighs heavily
on them. They are serious, a bit detached, closed, and do not show
their feelings much because they are working too hard. They have a
strong sense of right and wrong and can be critical of themselves
(and of others who do not live up to their own standards). They can
be a bit of the 'critical parent' type if they are not careful, getting a
little self-righteous and resentful if they do not feel appreciated.

In a sense they put too much into whatever they are engaged in
in their lives, they over-invest emotionally, over-identifying with
their cause and then becoming totally devastated if they lose. If the
business fails or the job is lost, if the beloved wife or husband leaves
or the child rebels, it is then that extreme anxiety, deep despair and
suicidal thoughts will begin to show themselves: after a shock, after
a profound loss, after prolonged responsibility they blame them-

selves for having neglected their duty and think they are unfit to live. They feel they could have done more, loved more, foreseen more.

Sufferers fall into the deepest kind of depression – an absolutely solid, stable, immovable depression blocking out everything else in life. They may still get on with life, keeping up the facade and going through the motions, but all feelings will have died, nothing can reassure or console them; there is no hope, they can see no light whatsoever at the end of the tunnel. They are in a pit, their depression is absolute and pervasive. They are quietly desperate.

They condemn themselves for failing. There is always deep self-condemnation inside the *Aurum* depression. If they are religious then they may believe that what has happened to them is the will of God. They may begin to feel that they have endangered their soul: they feel deep guilt and are haunted and tormented; they consider themselves bad, worthless. They are so depressed that nothing helps. They become suicidal, or get suicidal thoughts: they may dwell on suicide, planning it carefully, or they may impulsively jump from a height or crash the car.

At this stage of things they may also be irritable and irascible, even quarrelsome. They get angry easily, have outbursts of temper over nothing at all and easily take offence, thinking their friends are against them. They cannot bear to be contradicted. They get angry if their depression is intruded upon. They blame themselves for everything, and their only relief from this is to rage angrily at 'circumstances' and 'fate'.

There is also a lot of restlessness and anxiety in this psychological picture. *Aurum* is well indicated in anxiety states, especially when these centre on health matters (particularly worries about heart disease). The typical *Aurum* personality types are also often anxious about whether they have done wrong, have neglected their duty or have risked losing salvation. They are generally fearful and apprehensive, begin to develop fears of all kinds, such as a fear of going out (agoraphobia), of heights, of the dark.

Night-time is terrible for such people: *Aurum* is a remedy for the most fixed insomnia or restless sleep; for the relief of frightful dreams about thieves; for those who scream loudly while asleep or who dream of falling from a great height.

You'll often see the remedy in the sufferer's face, which can look bloated and red. There may be congestion of blood to the face and head or congestive flushing in the head and chest. The nose may be red (a typical 'drinker's nose' with a knobby tip) and reddened skin may peel off the nose and the face generally.

General and Characteristic Physical Symptoms

- Unbearable, boring pains which are worse at night and when too warm in bed. These are often associated with rheumatism or arthritis, but could also arise for no particular reason.
- Severe bone pain which wanders from site to site and disturbs sleep, sometimes driving the sufferer from bed in search of relief despite the fact that the pains are aggravated by movement. The small bones are often affected (such as those in the ears, nose and toes).
- A headache in the inside corner of the right eye, as well as chronic nasal obstruction and sinusitis, malignancy in the nose.
- The heart and circulation are often affected. Those affected may feel that their heart has skipped a beat, or as if it were standing still. Palpitations are common, as well as angina pectoris. Sufferers may develop high blood-pressure or suffer a heart attack or stroke.
- Sufferers may feel ravenous hunger or a complete loss of appetite; or suffer chronic indigestion or bilious disorders. They will be thirsty for cold drinks.
- Alcoholism or other drug abuse is a strong possibility in this remedy picture.
- A chilly constitution. Sufferers like to be wrapped up, but may still like fresh air.

States and conditions are improved by: moving, walking in the open or in the sunshine, warm air, summer, listening to classical music, in the evening.

States and conditions are made worse by: cloudy weather, dark gloomy days, sunset, midnight–2 or 3 a.m., morning, cold, pain, or any external impressions, winter, before menstruating.

States and conditions may be caused by: excessive drinking, grief, fright, disappointed love, financial loss, business reversal, prolonged anxiety, unusual responsibilities, severe emotional stress.

CALCAREA CARBONICA

(Calcium carbonate)

EMOTIONAL AND PSYCHOLOGICAL CHARACTERISTICS
Calcarea carbonica is made from the middle layer of the oyster shell, which is formed from the secretions of the oyster itself to provide protection and structure to the vulnerable and flabby creature within it. The person who needs this remedy is physically soft and flabby and emotionally vulnerable, full of fears and anxieties. She provides her own structure by developing a lifestyle which is methodical, practical, organized and controlled in order to conceal and shelter her inner vulnerability. Her tightly closed shell covers up the anxiety and vulnerability inside.

The person who needs *Calcarea carbonica* on a constitutional level is likely to have been a late developer (physically, mentally or both) as a child, and this in some cases may be the cause of her never feeling quite up to scratch, never quite equal to life, never being quite sure of herself or developing the confidence that she will be able to handle whatever turns up. In later life she may tend to be overweight, subject to glandular problems and generally to lack physical and mental energy.

Because she knows she has a limited amount of energy she plans very carefully, ordering her life so that she can do all she wants without overtiring herself. She is well organized, practical, methodical and hard-working (often a workaholic). She works to overcome her feelings of being inadequate physically and mentally, covering up her fundamental lack of self-confidence and timidity by achieving a level of often considerable competence through hard work. She protects herself from any potential criticism by working harder and harder, disguises her inner anxieties by pressing on, always anticipating and heading off criticism by being ever more conscientious. She can often seem completely impervious to outside opinion because when in doubt or under threat (real or imagined) she shuts up and closes down like an oyster, becoming completely unresponsive in order to conceal her internal anxiety. She always conceals her inner feelings, is very closed by nature, and can seem indifferent.

She works hard and effectively but cannot be hurried. She can become very obstinate out of a need to do things her own way and at her own pace in order not to get flustered and become unable to function, as she sees it. She will eventually take on too much, feel over-responsible, and will gradually wear herself out. Under too much stress, unable to continue her hard work and therefore to keep anxiety at bay, she will begin to tire and fear collapse. She may become sleepless with worry and then be unable to work properly the next day; she will think about all the things she has to do and worry about what will happen if she cannot do them. Her mind will race, she will get so tired that she cannot sleep, then, waking unrefreshed, she will worry even more that she will not be able to function if she is tired.

At this point others may begin to see her underlying fearful nature. Characteristically the *Calcarea* personality is full of fears and anxieties (it is one of the most anxious and fretful remedies in the **Materia Medica**). She suffers terribly from many phobias: about failing, not accomplishing; about disease and her health generally (she has a mania for reading medical books); about insects, heights, driving (or especially of being driven), thunderstorms, poverty, bad news, open spaces, closed spaces, people, the dark, being alone; about 'she scarcely knows what' – and she suffers from a growing fear of impending insanity. These fears are all the more terrible for not being apparent. She continues to function well while increasingly covering up her fears.

She is deeply self-conscious and profoundly afraid of what people will think about her. She hates being looked at and thinks people are watching her, maybe laughing at her. This fear arises from her conviction that if people observe her they will realize that she cannot really cope. At its deepest she fears that someone will notice her confusion and think her insane.

When this person's health breaks down you may see one of two pictures: she may slow right down, seemingly listless, apathetic and lazy, tired by the slightest physical or mental effort, easily discouraged, easily depressed and increasingly fearful, despairing of recovery. She may develop deeper fears: of dying, of spirits and ghosts; she may even develop delusions of evil things, spirits, demons; deep fears of the unknown emerge. On the other hand, you may witness a far more agitated personality: over-sensitive, jumpy, easily startled, irritable, excited by trifles, open to all sorts of external impressions, exceedingly distressed at hearing of cruelty, scared at the sight of wounds, feeling the impulse to scream or cry without apparent reason, breaking down in spells of 'causeless weeping'. Her sleep can be disturbed by terrifying dreams; she often has difficulty going to sleep because of the constant flow of anxious thoughts; she can lie awake till 2, 3, or 4 a.m.

This state is commonly seen in children, but in their case, of course, there is not usually a preceding period of over-responsibility. In children the state may be associated with teething or some food sensitivity or allergy.

General and Characteristic Physical Symptoms

- Weakness, easily fatigued.
- Flabby tissues, a tendency to put on weight (but can be thin).
- Poor circulation. Chilly and sensitive to cold and damp.
- Sweating easily (often a cold sweat). The typical sufferer has a 'wet fish' handshake. Children (and sometimes adults) sweat profusely around the head and scalp.
- Slow development as a child, with a tendency to catch colds and to get sore throats, tonsillitis and illnesses involving the glands.
- In later life sufferers are prone to the development of new growths (polyps, bony growths).
- The typical sufferer craves indigestible foods such as coal, chalk and raw potatoes. She may also crave eggs, sweet things and ice-cream. She either desires or detests milk (her digestion is

worse for milk in either case). She often feels hungry and her thirst may be marked.

- Arthritis, diabetes, hypertension, gall-bladder problems and gout are common illnesses in persons of this constitution.

States and conditions are improved by: dry weather, being constipated.

States and conditions are made worse by: cold of all kinds, intellectual or physical effort, the full moon.

States and conditions may be caused by: malnutrition (lack of calcium), fear, cold.

GELSEMIUM SEMPERVIRENS

(*Yellow jasmine*)

EMOTIONAL AND PSYCHOLOGICAL CHARACTERISTICS
Most people become familiar with *Gelsemium* first as a flu remedy, and indeed the most characteristic state of *Gelsemium* is the exhaustion that accompanies or follows a bout of flu: weakness, tiredness, apathy, a feeling of being completely drained of all energy or interest, a state of relaxation and weakness almost amounting to paralysis, when the body feels heavy, arms and legs feel like lead, and any exertion causes trembling. Just as this plant, a woody climber, needs to be supported on a frame lest it collapse, so the person needing *Gelsemium* needs support or will wilt and collapse.

Anxiety is felt severely: anyone needing this remedy will be very apprehensive about many things: death, crowds, wide open spaces, falling, exams, any engagements, public appearances, performances. In anxiety this characteristic *Gelsemium* state will come on: the person will shake, tremble and seize up, becoming paralysed, heavy and sluggish. He may be unable to speak; he may get diarrhoea. Nervous diarrhoea may come on as a result of stress, worry or anxiety. Or he may get heartburn and colic from stress and anxiety. Sufferers are in a constant state of anticipatory anxiety, fearing failure and/or that something bad is imminent.

This state can come on after an infection (commonly flu or glandular fever) or it may be associated with a weakened immune system following repeated infections. It may also come on after fear, shock, embarrassment, over-excitement or fright. It is a useful remedy in all cases of acute anticipatory anxiety, such as before taking a driving test, visiting the dentist, or for children who are nervous about going to school.

There is also a sluggish depression associated with this remedy. Sufferers want to be left alone, want to be quiet, but at the same time hate isolation. Such depression typically comes on after receiving bad news. They suffer from cloudiness of mind, unable to think or really concentrate; they become forgetful. *Gelsemium* can be helpful for people who have had a lot of infections and have become very weak and frail, with no confidence. It may be a good acute remedy for a person of a *Calcarea carbonica* constitution.

People needing this remedy are usually quite timid in general; their weakness makes them lose self-confidence, makes them frightened of taking on new projects or jobs in case they do not feel strong enough to complete them. They may even be afraid to leave the house. They find it difficult to express emotions.

There can be suicidal tendencies, with impulses to jump from heights.

General and Characteristic Physical Symptoms

- Nervous exhaustion. Weakness is particularly felt in the limbs, trembling from weakness is common and very characteristic. The weakness can even go as far as paralysis, especially of the legs and muscles. This remedy may be useful in MS and other neurological problems, as well as for ME (post-viral syndrome).
- Feverish states, with chills and a flushed face; internal chills as if ice-cold water had been poured down the sufferer's back.
- Headaches at the back and bottom of the head (occipital).
- Dullness and blurring of the vision, sometimes double vision.
- There are no strong food cravings, and no sense of thirst.

States and conditions are improved by: movement, sweating.

States and conditions are made worse by: heat, hot weather, bad news, excitement, anticipation.

States and conditions may be caused by: anticipation, fear of failure, viral infection, fright, fear, worry, exams, grief, excitement, shock, glandular fever, stage fright, performance anxiety.

IGNATIA AMARA

(Strychnos ignatia: St Ignatius' bean)

EMOTIONAL AND PSYCHOLOGICAL CHARACTERISTICS

Ignatia is the first remedy to think of when someone, male or female, is very upset, beside him- or herself, 'hysterical'. The distress may be caused by anything at all but is most often brought on by grief or bad news. *Ignatia* calms us down when we suddenly lose it, can't keep control: we may find ourselves weeping and laughing alternately or may be controlling our tears but letting out big sighs.

Its major acute use is for the effects of and reactions to grief, or separation from a lover or loved spouse ('disappointed love', as the old books put it). This is because we are nearly all thrown into an *Ignatia* state by death or the break-up of relationship, especially in the first stages of loss: we alternate between controlling our emotions with difficulty then releasing them in a rush, laughing and crying by turns, behaving irrationally, screaming and crying and then lapsing into numbed silence. This picture may also be seen in reaction to any shock or fright: being bitten by a dog, perhaps, or being attacked violently on the street or raped; also in the case of any fear, anger or anxiety.

It is also a remedy for people in whose lives grief or loss, and the failure to resolve them, has become a chronic feature for whatever reason. If the person doesn't get over such things appropriately: if they throw her off-balance long-term, causing her a general loss of confidence, then she needs *Ignatia*. There may be a 'loss of nerve', general fearfulness, a feeling that all is lost. The sufferer will also be inconsolable, and is made worse by attempts to console her.

There are also people who conform to the picture of *Ignatia* constitutionally. These people tend to be by nature sensitive and excitable, emotional, moody, to have what are now called 'histrionic' rather than hysterical personalities. They are easily melancholy and tearful, and disposed to mull over thoughts and problems.

In the chronic or constitutional picture you may not so often see the overtly excitable behaviour but more likely will witness a highly-strung, tautly-controlled individual, who may at first seem as reserved as the *Natrum muriaticum* type: the difference will be that in *Natrum muriaticum* the reserve will be all you do see, in *Ignatia* you may constantly get the feeling that this person, apparently silent and reserved, may suddenly burst out in emotions, is only just keeping herself under control. The control may be maintained while there are observers, but when alone or at night she may get upset, become sleepless, cry, not able to eat, sob, laugh out loud. A root issue in people with such natures may be that they are idealists, romantics: they are people who expect a lot from themselves and from life and are consequently constantly disappointed and frustrated by the realities of the world. Their constant disappointment may make them morose, bitter, critical, irritably perfectionist. They don't gradually become more realistic and practical as they observe the imperfections of the world, but persist in holding on to their ideal of how everything should be, continually wanting things to be the way they rarely can be – thus such people are continually disappointed.

These personalities are very hypersensitive: bad news can bring *Ignatia* out acutely, for instance in a migraine. It is also helpful to counter the effects of (even pleasurable) stress: plays, events – any activity involving concentrated nervous or physical strain can lead to a collapse requiring *Ignatia*.

Dread, fear and anxiety also run through the remedy. Much of the anxiety revolves around feelings of being trapped or constricted and being unable to break out. There may be emotional strain from having to stay in a marriage or a job that isn't working, isn't ideal, having to live a lie, or from living some other kind of false life – wherever there is the familiar *Ignatia* conflict caused by discrepancy between the ideal and the reality. Associated with this are fears of being trapped, of being possessed, of being changed. There is also the fear of insanity.

Irritability and anger can also feature in the *Ignatia* personality. She can be irritable with herself, sharp and critical towards others when upset: she sees the flaws in other people and 'has to' mention them. She may often seem like the *Nux vomica* type – irritable, over-sensitive, irascible, fault-finding, quarrelsome and accusing – but this is usually a product of being upset or disillusioned, perhaps because her high standards have not been met.

Sleep is often difficult: sufferers can dream all night of the same subject, dreams that are full of disappointment and failed expectations and efforts. There is also a strong tendency for dreams of water and of drowning. *Ignatia* is useful for the insomnia that can accompany grief, but it is also one of the remedies for extreme fatigue after grief, for those who want to sleep through their depression.

General and Characteristic Physical Symptoms

- Any physical symptoms that come on in the wake of high emotion or upset, such as headache, migraine, nausea, fainting, cough, colic.
- Spasmodic complaints such as twitching, jerking of muscles; spastic colon; hiccoughs; spasmodic cough.
- Fleeting, erratic pains.
- Temporary paralysis or numbness without apparent physical cause, such as paralysis of the vocal chords or tingling down one side of the body.
- General over-sensitivity to smells (especially tobacco), pain, and noise.
- Frequent, deep sighing.
- Frequent yawning.
- Sensation of a lump in the throat (*globus hystericus*).
- Paradoxical symptoms, such as indigestion which improves after eating; pain in the throat that is worse for liquids but not for solid food; hunger that is not relieved by eating; pain that is better for pressure.

States and conditions are improved by: socializing, having a good time, exposure to heat.

States and conditions are made worse by: mornings (especially around 11 a.m.), unpleasant emotions, consolation, strong smells (tobacco, coffee, etc.).

States and conditions may be caused by: grief, emotional shock, fear, fright, vexation, emotional worry, bottled-up anger, held-back indignation, accidents, disappointment in love.

LACHESIS

(Lachesis trigonocephalus; Venom of the Surukuku or Bushmaster snake)

EMOTIONAL AND PSYCHOLOGICAL CHARACTERISTICS
This is a remedy for people of a passionate nature, for those who get heavily involved in whatever they are concerned with and who are passionately intense about things. Their moods and behaviour characteristically alternate between periods of excitement and depression. This alternation might appear merely to take the form of mood swings, or you may see it in its most intense form, i.e. manic-depressive illness. The cycle can take place daily with, for example, sadness in the morning and excitement in the evening, or there can be more prolonged periods in each state. Sometimes the depression seems to be caused by exhaustion following on from the energetic state.

In the up phase of the cycle the person who needs *Lachesis* may be intense, energetic, self-confident, enthusiastic, excitable and enormously articulate and talkative. He may be full of ideas and conviction, talking very quickly, fascinating like the snake.

In the down phase of the cycle there will be periods of depression, restless anxiety and even silence; or the talkativeness may become rambling incoherence. Suspicion, jealousy and spitefulness may emerge: the person may imagine that he is being cheated, talked about, hated and plotted against and, like the snake, he may strike first. *Lachesis* is revengeful. The eyes are often the tell-tale sign that a person needs *Lachesis*: they may look like snake's eyes, flickering from beneath heavy lids.

Material from the unconscious (so-called shadow material) is never far from the surface in the *Lachesis* personality. The subject is often very sensitive, even psychic; he commonly has disturbing dreams: of ghosts, the dead, funerals and coffins. Sleeping can feel dangerous because of the release of unconscious material; the person may jerk awake when dropping off to sleep. He is easily affected by alcohol, which also allows material to erupt from the unconscious. Sexuality, too, is a strongly developed area of expression – if it is blocked there can be problems: anxiety, restlessness or irritability, for example.

The *Lachesis* personality is well and fully functioning as long as he can express himself, discharge his strong feelings, ideas, plans, his sexuality. He is ill when this expression is blocked for whatever reason. When hurt he gets angry, on the whole, not withdrawn; he becomes revengeful, not broody; malicious, not self-blaming. When he grieves he does so with anger and a desire for revenge. There is always vitality and usually extraversion.

Despite this extravert self-presentation a very low self-esteem lies at the root of a lot of *Lachesis* symptoms. The person needs to be acknowledged as exceptional, as special, otherwise he may be extremely negative and take revenge, behaving maliciously and vindictively. His self-centredness, possessiveness and jealousy all have their origin in his deep fear of not being good enough. He cannot stand being limited, controlled or constricted.

Lachesis may be highly indicated for some types of manic depression, for schizophrenia, or for deep mental and emotional problems. The full picture may only emerge under the influence of alcohol for some people. It is one of the main remedies for alcoholism.

A sufferer's characteristic fears are strongly related to his suspiciousness: fear of robbers, that someone is going to come into the house and steal something, that someone will hurt them. He thinks someone will stab him in the back; he fears someone lurking behind him. He gets claustrophobia, is apprehensive about the future, and worries about his heart and blood-pressure. This suspiciousness can lead him to become critical and fault-finding.

Characteristically very loquacious and animated, with an overactive mind and imagination, this person, if religious, may develop fears about religion: that his friends are possessed by the devil, that he himself is persecuted, that Satan is after him trying to tempt him.

He is frightened of becoming possessed, and develops a fear of a superhuman power overtaking him. In short, a strong sense of paranoia, a conviction that everyone is out to get him, is a hallmark of this state.

General and Characteristic Physical Symptoms

- Everything may be worse after sleep, on waking.
- Symptoms may be focused, or may begin, down the left-hand side of the body, perhaps then moving to the right-hand side.
- There is extreme hypersensitivity: the sufferer is sensitive to light, noise, light touch, heat.
- Inability to bear constriction round throat or abdomen.
- Better for discharge of any kind: body fluids, start of menstruation.
- Warm-bloodedness; sufferers are badly affected in stuffy rooms or by heat generally. Problems of blood circulation: it is known as a bleeding remedy, important in heart complaints and to moderate blood-pressure.
- Hormonal imbalance in women, especially PMS and the menopause.

States and conditions are improved by: discharges, start of a period, moderate temperatures, fresh air.

States and conditions are made worse by: delayed or suppressed discharges, constriction, sun, heat generally, being touched, after sleep, the Spring.

States and conditions may be caused by: menopause, alcoholism, grief, rejection.

LYCOPODIUM CLAVATUM

(Wolf's claw, Club moss)

EMOTIONAL AND PSYCHOLOGICAL CHARACTERISTICS
This is a prickly-leaved plant which creeps along the ground, root-
ing itself at intervals. Its fruit contains spores that yield a powder
which burns with a quick flare when thrown into a flame. The
fundamental characteristic of people who need *Lycopodium* is often
the combination of lack of confidence in themselves and authori-
tarian behaviour – the very combination represented in the plant's
trademarks of ground-creeping, prickliness and tendency to flare up.
In the *Lycopodium* personality there is frequently a mixture of
cowardice and arrogance, timidity and authority, an interplay
continually and varyingly represented in their behaviour and their
lives.

In the acute stage such people suffer markedly from anticipatory
anxiety, panicking before making any kind of public appearance,
giving talks or taking exams. However, once started, they always
perform well and with authority: they perform well because they
prepare well, work hard. Their diffidence and lack of self-
confidence, however, their fear of being found out, makes the
prospect of a public appearance terrifying.

They are generally very fearful and subject to panics, though this
is not always obvious because they avoid at all costs situations which
give rise to them. They fear crowds, closed places (claustrophobia),
going out of the house (agoraphobia), the dark, illness (a real
hypochondriasis) and death. Many of their fears are clearly related to
their fundamental lack of self-esteem: the fear of failure, fear that

they will not reach their destination, fear of being found out, fear of exposure, fear of nervous breakdown, fear of undertaking anything, fear of dying.

To protect themselves against these fears they develop competence in certain well-defined areas, often academic, avoiding emotion, and become the experts in their own (narrow) field, in areas where no one can match them, or where they can acquire sufficient mastery of their material to remain substantially unchallenged. They are conscientious and orderly in a quiet sort of way. They know they cannot cope with contradiction and challenge, and so avoid any occasions where these might arise.

It is when these tactics do not work and they are actually confronted that we see the other side of their character: they may become angry, blustering and openly tyrannical, or may make an ignominious and speedy retreat. They can be quite calm and likeable, if a little detached, outside the home, but within it they can be tyrants – in a subtle way, to be sure, but their word at home is law. Even their tyranny will be understated and calm, though it is likely to be pushed into more active mode by teenage children when they begin to rebel.

Outbursts of temper are characteristic but surprising. They take offence quickly, dwell on resentments, explode suddenly in anger. They can also get extremely depressed, feel in despair on waking in the morning, get as far down as to feel really tired of life. They try to avoid softer emotions and feelings: emotions can get out of control, leaving them vulnerable to others. There is always a certain detachment, often experienced as superiority, haughtiness, in the *Lycopodium* profile. Nevertheless they like to be liked and can be quite charming when they want to be.

They enjoy sexual relationships, too, and can be amorous. However, they have difficulty trusting themselves in relationships, especially long-term ones, fearing both rejection and commitment. They may get out of relationships just when it looks as if they are settling down to something permanent. They are afraid of being completely alone, however, so seek relationships which don't tie them, summed up by the expression 'likes to be alone, with someone in the next room'.

They may have a sentimental streak which seems at odds with

their aloofness; they can be both sympathetic and affectionate. They weep over sentimental scenes, are nostalgic, weep when thanked.

Timidity and fear make them cautious: they can be miserly with money, fearful of change or of not being able to support themselves or their family. They are not at all passionate and can seem very dry.

The characteristic lack of self-confidence is associated with a lot of psychosexual problems in men: they may suffer a decrease in sexual desire or potency; anticipatory fears of inadequacy may affect them: they may be unable to sustain erections, or may suffer from premature ejaculation.

Never very physically robust, as they age they become even less so and can, indeed, become prematurely old, with a tendency to dry, wrinkled skin and greying hair and the characteristic lined forehead. They may also suffer premature memory loss and mental confusion.

General and Characteristic Physical Symptoms

- Symptoms are markedly on the right-hand side of the body, perhaps then extending to the left-hand side.
- Sufferers are chilly and hate the cold, but at the same time are wearied by great heat and oppressed by stuffy atmospheres.
- Many digestive symptoms: sufferers may be hungry but then feel full after a few mouthfuls; they become bloated and flatulent soon after eating but get no relief from passing wind or burping. Migraines that originate from digestive problems.
- Cravings for sugar, sweet things, hot foods and drinks. Intolerance of cabbage, beans, onions, oysters, pastry.
- Sufferers cannot stand clothes that are too tight around the waist.
- Respiratory problems; a tendency to catch colds, bronchitis, pneumonia.
- One foot is often hot, the other cold.
- General physical awkwardness and weakness, with poor muscle tone.

States and conditions are improved by: keeping busy, cool open air, hot foods and drinks, warmth, loose clothes.

States and conditions are made worse by: certain times of day or night (4–8 p.m., on waking), being contradicted, cold foods or drinks, hot stuffy atmospheres, emotional stress, worry.

States and conditions may be caused by: old age, chronic illness, menopause, premature senility, being bullied as a child.

NATRUM MURIATICUM

(Sodium chloride, salt)

EMOTIONAL AND PSYCHOLOGICAL CHARACTERISTICS
A person needing *Natrum muriaticum* is usually quiet and self-contained, a little self-conscious and awkward, reserved and rather introverted, perfectly pleasant but slightly on guard, wary of emotional involvement with others. She will be easy to talk to, a good listener, helpful, unobtrusive and sympathetic – but you will not get to know her easily. Even if she wanted to she would find it difficult to let someone through the wall she has built up over the years. She will help you but will not open up to you.

It is not that she is not emotional: she is capable of very deep emotions, but she fears being hurt more than anything and will not willingly make herself vulnerable. She will not easily let anyone near her emotionally, will try to avoid being in a position where someone might get attached to her; if she falls in love herself it will be with people who are 'unavailable'. It is not the attachment she fears but what she sees to be the inevitable end of the relationship: the loss and betrayal, the bereavement. One of her greatest fears and anxieties is that she will be robbed: she cannot bear the thought of having something taken from her without permission, of being broken into, betrayed.

Another way she protects herself is by living in the past. She seems to hang on to past disappointments and hurts, painful memories and resentments. She is haunted by unpleasant thoughts about the past, about how she has been wronged. She bears grudges against anyone who has offended her. Because of what happened in the past she will never risk being hurt again. If she is bereaved she will find it difficult to resolve her grief because there is a part of her that wants to hang on to it. Hanging on to the past protects her from the present.

Because of her fear of emotional attachment she can often be a very lonely person. To some extent this is her choice: she likes to be alone – but she is also afraid of loneliness. She wants a relationship but only one which is deep and meaningful. If she cries she cries alone and does not like sympathy or consolation partly because she does not believe it is genuine or that people really understand. She has a strong aversion to sympathy or consolation and may become angry or tearful if either is offered.

Her emotions may leak out despite herself, sometimes seeming inappropriate: she may laugh uncontrollably at something sad or serious, cry while laughing or cry a great deal over what appear to others to be trifles. Laughter is an important mode of expression: she specializes in gallows humour. She may be cheerful and sad in quick succession. She may overreact to a small thing and get suddenly and surprisingly angry, while other, apparently worse things may have aroused no response in her.

There are a lot of similarities between this remedy picture and that of *Ignatia*. The personality of *Natrum muriaticum* can appear quite contradictory and variable: she can oscillate between excitement and despondency, assertiveness and diffidence, robustness and weakness. She can be impulsive where she is normally orderly and contained; she can have unexpected rages and hates.

The fear of being hurt extends beyond her own personality: she cannot bear others being hurt either. She feels for the sufferings of the world, rather than for herself. Disguising her own pain in that of others, she adopts an idealistic defence against her own emotions, crying for others but finding it difficult to cry for herself. Her tears come only after long restraint and a brave effort to hold them back and carry on alone.

She is very fearful and suffers from many complaints as a result. Fear of robbers is strong and symbolic for her. She is often afraid of insects. She suffers from claustrophobia, a fear of heights, fear of the dark. She has deep fears of losing control, of being ridiculed or laughed at, made a fool of.

She also descends into deep depression from time to time, often too deep for her to be able to acknowledge it. Loathing of life and a desire for death is very strong, though this seems to remain passive. Suicidal thoughts or attempts at suicide are not present; it is rather that she wishes she could be dead. She is really quite pessimistic, believing that if things are going right they will soon go wrong. The depression may arise from her deep sense of guilt: she is always ready to feel guilt and remorse, to blame herself. It may also arise from suppressed anger: she has no mechanism for expressing personal anger efficiently, she either feels angry on behalf of others or the world, or she fails to express it and broods resentfully over past wrongs without ever voicing these feelings, or else lashing out about something completely different.

Natrum muriaticum is one of the major remedies used for profound weakness and emotional breakdown that arise from too much or too prolonged stress. This is partly because of this personality type's seemingly endless capacity to absorb distress: eventually the failure to react takes its toll, often in a physical form. Much of her suppressed emotion may find expression through the body in illness or fear of illness: the ultimate loss of self-control. She is very hypochondriacal, and is always actively looking to be healthy like *Arsenicum*.

General and Characteristic Physical Symptoms

- Physical characteristics: thin, pale-skinned, prone to herpes (cold sores) on the lips, a lower lip that is often cracked vertically down the middle.
- Disturbed fluid balance: the sufferer may easily retain water and other bodily fluids in several different forms, such as generalized oedema (water-retention), pre-menstrual syndrome, severe constipation, mucus formation, greasy hair and skin, headaches. Or she may suffer from excessive dryness of skin and hair, lose a lot of bodily fluids and look scrawny.
- Sensitivity to cold.
- A good appetite, intense thirst (for water or tea).
- Sufferers may crave (or hate) salt and salty foods, bread, or may have a strong dislike (intolerance) of bread and sometimes salt.
- Exhaustion that comes on after only little effort.

- Over-acute senses, especially hearing. In particular, sufferers may be hypersensitive to sudden or scratchy noises, and to music, which may either please or irritate.
- Inability to urinate in public.

States and conditions are improved by: open air, not eating, being at the seaside.

States and conditions are made worse by: consolation, certain times of the morning (particularly 10 a.m.), being at the seaside (although as mentioned above this can also improve conditions for some sufferers), intellectual work, direct heat, sun, full moon, extremes of temperature, stress, over-excitement.

States and conditions may be caused by: emotional sensitivity, shock, a history of malaria, quinine.

NUX VOMICA

(Poison nut; Vomiting nut)

EMOTIONAL AND PSYCHOLOGICAL CHARACTERISTICS
This remedy is derived from a nut which is the main source of the
poison strychnine. Overdoses of strychnine cause very difficult
breathing, unbearable anxiety, twitching, spasm and convulsions as
well as exaggerated sensitivity to all external stimuli. Think of *Nux
vomica* whenever you see a person who is very alive, responsive,
active and engaged. He may also be tense, impatient, irritable,
competitive, doing everything quickly, always just about to move on
to the next thing – or perhaps he used to be like this before he
became exhausted and ill.

This remedy may be indicated constitutionally – that is, the
person may be more or less like this the whole of his life, in sickness or
in health – or he may temporarily be in a state of needing it,
perhaps as a result of taking too many drugs, drinking too much, or
being generally stressed from overwork. *Nux vomica* is useful for the
state that used to be called 'liverish', and indeed the symptoms are often
brought about by the liver being overloaded with alcohol. It tends to
be associated with the type of person who eats, drinks or smokes too
much, stays up too late and is generally over-excitable. In short, think
of *Nux vomica* where there is excess of any kind of appetite.

The main thing you will be aware of with a person in a *Nux
vomica* state is his edgy, excitable, aggressive energy. This may
express itself in hard work and hard living – a full, active, lifestyle –
or in irritability, bad temper and anger (or a mixture of both!). The
person who needs this remedy is someone who can easily pick

quarrels or start a fight; he feels better after expressing some of his irritability and frustration in this way.

He is impatient, always in a hurry, punctual and anxious not to waste time. He gets frustrated quickly if things do not go right the first time; he is exasperated with others' slowness and tends to be critical and fault-finding with those less competent than himself. Perfectionist and orderly, he does not like disorder. He is quite fussy over little things.

He is always trying to push himself beyond what his system can cope with. He always wants to do more than he can, both emotionally and physically. He appears to be very self-confident and decisive, never talking about his worries or doubts and acting quickly to resolve tension (sometimes too impulsively). Nothing satisfies him and any failure is experienced as humiliation – his pride is easily wounded. He cannot cope with criticism, contradiction or any obstacles being put in his way, nor with anything that holds him up.

However, underlying his great drive is anxiety about many things: work, the future, financial and physical security, health. These anxieties will not paralyse him, but will push him to try and sort them out, overcome them. If he cannot overcome them by hard work then he may become exhausted and depleted, may suffer from insomnia (either because he cannot sleep for the rush of ideas that come, or for being upset), or he may fall asleep but wake anxious early in the morning (characteristically at 3 a.m.). Then there may come depression, even suicidal thoughts: *Nux vomica* is one of the main remedies for suicidal thoughts. This type of personality, however, rarely actually commits suicide.

He is emotionally sensitive, touchy and quick to take offence, reacting to the slightest criticism, contradiction or imagined insult. His emotions are very near to the surface, are quickly expressed and then quickly subside: he is impulsively angry, irritable, kind, generous, sympathetic, sentimental. He is moody, but in the sense of being irritable rather than weepy. He is particularly strongly affected by failure to achieve his ambitions or by wounded honour. He is capable of being malicious and taking revenge and can even have sudden impulses to violence. He has a fear of knives, and may feel the impulse to kill when he sees a sharp knife.

As you might expect, this kind of person finds it difficult to relax and will be likely to use drugs and stimulants to keep going. This may begin with a mild tranquillizer or a drink in the evening and then develop into a spiral of addiction which ends in exhaustion and depletion of his vital energies.

General and Characteristic Physical Symptoms

- Cravings for alcohol, spicy foods, fats, condiments and coffee.
- Digestive problems: sufferers have a lot of indigestion and tend towards constipation (wants to but can't) and piles. Biliousness is a keynote.
- Sensitivity to cold, but a dislike of stuffy atmospheres.
- Hatred of wind and edginess before thunderstorms.
- Spasmodic conditions: nervous twitches, spasmodic movements; spasmodic sneezing on waking.
- Over-sensitive nervous system: sufferers react sharply and quickly to cold, bright light, even the slightest noise, various smells, environmental influences, pollens etc. These sensitivities often develop into allergic reactions.
- Unbearable shooting, tearing or stitching pains.
- Addictions: *Nux vomica* is extremely useful in the early stages of withdrawal from any addiction: its symptoms resemble the characteristic withdrawal symptoms: anxiety, tension, irritability, muscle spasm, hypersensitivity to one's environment, sleeplessness.

States and conditions are improved by: sleep, heat, night, wet weather.

States and conditions are made worse by: morning (on waking and between 3 and 4 a.m.), cold, cold dry weather, wind, stimulants. Symptoms are also more severe after meals.

States and conditions may be caused by: overuse of stimulants (including coffee, tea and tobacco) or tranquillizers, alcohol, a sedentary life, prolonged mental or emotional strain.

PHOSPHORUS

(The metal: White phosphorus)

EMOTIONAL AND PSYCHOLOGICAL CHARACTERISTICS
The metal phosphorus produces light without heat and bursts
spontaneously into flames unless it is kept under water. Its name
means carrier or conveyor of light. This is an excellent image for the
strongest characteristic of the *Phosphorus* remedy picture: diffuse
brightness without depth.

The person needing *Phosphorus* is sensitive, enthusiastic, outgoing
and gregarious. She needs people around in order to feel well and
happy, needs close physical (even sexual) contact and intimacy,
needs attention and reassurance and can become quite withdrawn if
her affection and openness are not returned, leaving her feeling
empty, alone and without identity. She is generous as well, offering
as well as receiving affection and support.

She lives very much in the moment, is very impressionable and
hypersensitive to everything around her: to light, noise, smells, but
especially to emotional atmospheres. She is a psychic sponge, soak-
ing up all the impressions that invade and bombard her from the
external world, or even from other worlds, for the spirit world may
seem as real to her as everyday life. She may take for granted the
presence of ghosts or spirits, have prophetic dreams, 'know' when
those she loves are ill or distressed.

She is sympathetic and can even be over-sympathetic, identifying
with the feelings, thoughts and interests of others to such an extent
as to lose any sense of her separate identity. She gets drawn into
identification with others, with suffering; she cannot maintain her

own boundaries. She is easily enthusiastic and interested in many things, then becomes bored or loses energy. She is an intuitive thinker with a short attention span, moving quickly from one interest and one person to another, not liking to be limited or trapped in one place. This may lead to her being productive only fitfully, and to have difficulty finishing things or really getting to grips with anything.

She can be very up and down emotionally, giving way to tantrums or outbursts of rage which are quickly over. Alternation between excitement and depression, between high energy and collapse is highly characteristic of this remedy picture, though much less so than with *Lachesis*, for example. Such an impressionable nature is very prone to depression. The *Phosphorus* down may be merely a natural reaction to the up, but the sufferer can also sink into a serious state of loathing of life, deep despondency, suicidal despair, sadness and dejection. She gets totally exhausted and unable to make any kind of effort. She can become irritable and apathetic and then does not want to think, talk or work.

The main cause or origin of all *Phosphorus* complaints is this general over-sensitivity. Because the person is highly impressionable and susceptible to her surroundings, disagreeable or unpleasant feelings can make her physically ill, bringing on trembling stomach and head pains, or palpitations. Even pleasant feelings can affect her like this.

She is easily startled and full of fears and anxieties. She is terrified of what may happen in the future, has deep fears of being alone (especially at twilight or at night when her imagination is at it most heightened); she is anxious about disease and death. She is afraid of thunder and lightning, of illness, of impending misfortune, of the future. These fears derive from her intense imagination and im-pressionability rather than from timidity. Her fearful state of mind can often cause insomnia; she sleeps unsoundly, has many anxious dreams and is subject to sleepwalking. She may get palpitations with fear and anxiety.

As an adult she may retain a childlike way of charming everyone – it is difficult for her not to please and entertain continually. Yet she loses the sense of her true self in constantly being available to others. In the end she may find little solidity in herself or in her achievements and may feel trapped in the role of entertainer, or else she may get so much appreciative feedback for her role that she may tend to overestimate herself, taking credit for achievement without actually putting in the necessary apprenticeship, becoming a true eternal child of the New Age. The survival issue for her is that she should be liked, and she is often tragically caught up in the attempt to please everyone all the time.

General and Characteristic Physical Symptoms

- Tall and slender; general lack of physical energy.
- Liver problems: hepatitis, cirrhosis.
- Heavy bleeding that begins easily: nosebleeds, menstrual bleeding, rectal bleeding; blood from the lungs, ulcers or gums.
- Burning sensations, especially in the palms of the hands.
- A craving for salt and salty foods, cold foods and drinks; an unquenchable thirst for cold water (but sufferers may feel nauseous when this water warms in the stomach). A strange desire to eat at 3 a.m.; an aversion to sweet foods, meat, tea, boiled milk, salted fish, oysters.

States and conditions are improved by: heat, sleep, eating.

States and conditions are made worse by: cold, storms, lying on the left side, twilight, walking quickly.

States and conditions may be caused by: over-rapid growth, loss of vital fluids, storms or lightning, excessive sexual activity.

PLATINUM METALLICUM

(The metal: Platinum)

EMOTIONAL AND PSYCHOLOGICAL CHARACTERISTICS
Platinum is one of the rarest and most precious of earth's metals: it
is cold and hard. The people who need it will appear to be cold and
hard too, regarding themselves as superior to all others. The most
characteristic symptoms of the remedy picture are pride, haughtiness, arrogance, contempt. People for whom it is useful behave in a
pompous and egotistical way and are frequently rude, scornful and
insulting to others. They are impatient and cannot stand being
contradicted. They may also dress to impress, either flashily or
elegantly. Sometimes this characteristic haughtiness and contempt
will not be so obvious: you could not actually swear it was there but
your experience is that you always feel inferior to these people and,
what's more important, you feel it is vital to them that you should
feel this way.

This apparent disdain arises out of their own anguished sense of
inadequacy. They feel so worthless that they have to keep themselves
separate from others. This side of *Platina* is revealed in the extensive fears, anxieties and sense of worthlessness and depression which
are a hidden part of the picture. While outwardly they appear
confident, imperiously sweeping all before them, inwardly they are
struggling against terrifying fears. Often these remain unconscious
and appear only in dreams or when they break down completely.

They fear, for example, that their partner or children will die, or
will simply not come home. They fear imminent death and have
premonitions about dying and see ghosts. The death they fear is

violent: being strangled, murdered, hanged. They suffer from anxiety about their health (fear of heart disease or of having a stroke). They even suffer from anxiety as a result of joyful things or excitement. When anxious they tend to be restless and excitable, walking about, trembling, their breathing constricted and suffering violent palpitations.

At the same time they may suffer from a compulsive desire to injure or kill those close to them, their children and the people they love most. These impulses can feel almost irresistible and they do not trust themselves around knives. It is as if they are terrified to be close to anyone, so they keep everyone at arm's length by acting in a superior way, or by feeling hostility. They also tend to be extremely jealous of others' success, which also serves to keep people at a distance.

Their out-of-touchness extends to the expression of emotion: people needing *Platina* often express what seems to others to be inappropriate emotions. They move from tears to laughter for no apparent reason; they can laugh at sad things and cry when there seems to be insufficient cause; they are irritable over trifles, are easily offended and can sulk for a long time.

Their depression can be marked, with suicidal tendencies. They come to loathe life, to feel that they have had enough of it. Their sense of being superior and separate becomes oppressive to them: they may experience themselves as being completely alone, deserted. They may come to feel that they don't belong anywhere, that they have no place in the world. If religion is part of their lives they may develop religious insanity, imagining that they have lost their chance of salvation, that they are separated from the saved. They may get intensely sad, blame themselves and threaten suicide.

Just as their fears and anxieties belie their public presentation, so their sleep also gives them away. It is frequently disturbed by dreams of sexual activity or fire, war and bloodshed. They may wake in the middle of the night with feelings of having left their bodies.

Eventually, there may be a breakdown. The feelings of being more important than others may overwhelm them, either temporarily or permanently: they can become trapped in the state labelled schizophrenia, feeling or having delusions that they are royalty or some famous, powerful person from history. They may have true delusions that everything is small, that everybody is mentally and physically inferior while they are large and superior.

On the other hand they may develop a mania in which their emotional lability might become even more exaggerated – in this case they may be found whistling, singing and dancing, talking constantly of things which are completely fanciful, or talking constantly of sexual matters.

Sexuality is normally a strong part of the *Platina* picture. Such personality types tend to be compulsively sexually preoccupied and active. They may have become sexually active early, or may have been involved with a lot of different people during their lives. Thus this may be a useful remedy where people feel *driven* to sexual promiscuity. Those who need *Platina* may lack the fundamental confidence to stay in a long-term relationship – and in any case their contemptuous behaviour may deter prospective partners. On the other hand this remedy may be useful for people whose sex drive has been suppressed. Sexuality, like other aspects of the *Platina* picture, is prone to be exaggerated or distorted.

General and Characteristic Physical Symptoms

- A sense of being bigger than others (physically as well as psychologically). Sufferers might experience the sensation, rather than the belief, that their body is larger than it is, that others are smaller than they are.
- 'Somatization': getting physical symptoms when emotionally disturbed. Often physical and emotional symptoms alternate.
- Numbness, often painful, in small spots on various parts of the body, especially on the head. Coldness in some body parts.
- Constrictive sensations, as if the limbs were bandaged.
- Cramping, spasmodic, shifting neuralgic pains.
- Trembling and tremulousness.
- Hypersensitivity of the genital area; also a tendency to genital itching and irritation, numbness and tingling sensations.
- Debility, fatigue and boredom.
- Lack of appetite or ravenousness; uncontrollable eating accompanied by feelings of self-hatred and/or hatred of others.
- Haemorrhage, especially in labour.
- Ovarian pain, cysts.

States and conditions are improved by: walking in the open air, eating.

States and conditions are made worse by: emotions, sex, touch, nervous exhaustion, fasting, evening.

States and conditions may be caused by: fright, excitement, disappointment, shock, sexual abuse, prolonged haemorrhaging, grief, wounded pride.

PULSATILLA NIGRICANS

(Wind flower, Meadow anemone)

EMOTIONAL AND PSYCHOLOGICAL CHARACTERISTICS
The pulsatilla is a small, pretty, purplish wildflower that does well on dry chalky or sandy soil, likes to grow in the company of other flowers, and is easily shaken by the wind and easily uprooted. It is small and delicate, with a flexible stem which bends one way or another according to the direction of the prevailing wind. There you have the essence of the *Pulsatilla* state or personality type.

The person needing *Pulsatilla* can be charming, agreeable, entertaining and pleasant in a quiet, mild sort of way. He is generally easily and openly emotional, can express feelings without embarrassment, will weep at sad films, cry easily and feel better for crying, be readily affectionate and touch and kiss easily. He will relate well to other people, enjoying their company and support. He does not like to quarrel or be in conflict with anyone so he is generally helpful, conciliatory and sensitive to others' feelings. He likes company and affection but is not so generous about giving his own, as is the *Phosphorus* personality type.

He will be reactive rather than proactive, easily influenced by others, readily taking on their opinions and perhaps becoming very indecisive for fear of causing offence. He likes to find out what will please others and is reluctant to offend or hurt them. He is always looking for someone or something stronger than he for support; he is generally dependent in nature.

This is the picture of an ordinary field-dependent person, the kind of person who quite simply and clearly enjoys company and support and will ask for it quite directly. People with this kind of personality nearly always get what they want by being pleasant and expressing their needs. *Pulsatilla* is often said to be a 'woman's remedy': it is true that women were once culturally conditioned to be like this more than men were, but these days it is probably no more a woman's remedy than a man's.

Usually such people are unaggressive, being more liable to blame themselves than others. However, they need a lot of open affection and reassurance and they can be touchy and easily hurt – they are very sensitive to criticism and can be surprisingly quick to take offence.

If they cannot get the attention they need by being pleasant they may become sullen and cross, uncommunicative and ill-humoured, discontented, capricious and peevish. They are easily hurt and discouraged. It is then that the selfishness of the remedy picture becomes apparent, then that malleability and dependency may become manipulation and demand. The person then expects others to care for him, feels unappreciated if they do not and can be jealous and possessive; his need for company may become excessive and demanding, and family and friends can feel trapped.

Give this remedy to anyone, man or woman, when you see this childlike neediness emerging inappropriately. It is useful whenever we are in the grip of that abandoned, miserable, clingy part of ourselves. Even in children it is useful if the child regresses to a dependency earlier than his years.

This personality type can become quite depressed if it comes about that he is genuinely alone and unsupported. Sadness, loneliness and self-pity emerge. Some of the most prominent fears in the remedy picture relate to loneliness, with fears of being alone (especially in the evening), of being abandoned, forsaken, helpless, unloved.

Jealousy is also a major symptom: in this remedy picture it originates in a desperate fear of abandonment. He may not always show his feelings: he may grieve inwardly and silently over some loss and he may have suicidal urges (specifically of drowning himself).

Pulsatilla also has a suspicious side: distrustful, anxious and hypochondriacal. He is timid and has many fears: of the dark, of ghosts, of crowds, of open spaces, of going insane, of illness, of impending domestic troubles. He can develop strange preoccupations and convictions – for instance that certain foods should not be eaten, that the opposite sex is dangerous – or may formulate religious ideas which can reach the stage of obsession. He may lie awake at night from worry with some single idea running obsessively through his mind.

Changeability is a strong feature of this emotional picture, probably largely because this person depends so much on others for his mood. He can be tender-hearted, easily hurt, responsive to kindness, easily discouraged, elated and/or depressed in quick succession.

The characteristic state with this, as with any remedy, may be there from early in life (a constitutional tendency), or it may be brought on as a result of circumstances: in this case the trigger might be the end of a relationship, especially the death of a mother or other very supportive person, or it might stem from having been abandoned as a child (even, in a vulnerable child, for just a few minutes). *Pulsatilla* is known as the remedy for the Inner Child: the part that has not grown up emotionally and feels unloved by his parents.

In this state of feeling unloved and abandoned this person may eat for comfort – this may lead to weight problems, even bulimia. He craves pastries, sweets, chocolate, and buttery, creamy foods.

General and Characteristic Physical Symptoms

- Changeableness and variability of all symptoms.
- Circulation is unstable; feelings of being hot and cold alternate (sufferers feel cold in a warm room and yet cannot bear to be anywhere too warm and stuffy); one part of the body may be hot, another cold; sufferers flush or blush easily.
- Energy levels vary: sufferers can pass quickly from being bright and lively to feeling tired and droopy.
- Pains are shifting and variable: in rheumatism the pains wander from one part of the body to another, shifting rapidly from joint to joint.
- Discharges are bland and creamy yellow or greeny-yellow.
- Sufferers are disposed to catarrhal conditions: long-lasting head

colds culminating in deafness; glue ear; earaches; rhinitis.
- Eye problems are common: agglutinated (in the mornings), conjunctivitis, styes.
- Menstrual periods tend to be delayed, scanty and painful; periods are easily stopped (due to anorexia, going abroad, upset). Puberty is a particularly difficult time.
- Tendency to varicose veins, chilblains, cold extremities.
- General lack of thirst.
- Sufferers crave butter, pastries, creamy foods and ice-cream – all of which disagree with them.
- Nausea, vomiting, heartburn all made worse by greasy, fried or rich fatty foods. Constipation and piles may occur.

States and conditions are improved by: gentle motion, fresh air, pregnancy, sympathy, consolation, company.

States and conditions are made worse by: being alone, evening, twilight, morning, heat, stuffy rooms, rich foods.

States and conditions may be caused by: abandonment, bereavement, change, loss of friends and familiar surroundings, sudden chill, getting wet.

SEPIA

(Cuttlefish/Squid ink)

EMOTIONAL AND PSYCHOLOGICAL CHARACTERISTICS
This blackish-brown inky liquid, secreted by the squid to conceal it
from danger or to camouflage it while it is attacking its prey, is an
apt image for the *Sepia* condition: the sufferer often seems to be
enveloped in a dark cloud of depression or indifference, from which
she occasionally emerges to make an attack. The person needing this
remedy may also look rather brownish, with her sallow skin,
tendency to develop age spots and brown discolorations of pigment,
and slight moustache.

Sepia is well known for its usefulness in the emotional distress
which can affect many women either pre-menstrually, in pregnancy,
after childbirth or during the menopause. Hormonal imbalance at
these times is a strong influence on the development of the remedy
picture. This is not to say that it is not helpful for men as well, and
for problems other than those caused by hormonal imbalance: the
symptoms are often brought on by exhaustion, for example.

The picture of this personality type while still functioning well and
before developing illness is that of a vital, hard-working person who
will take on anything. She has abundant energy, is full of life,
intelligent, assertive and direct. She is highly competent, at work or
in running a family, and sees no reason why she should apologize for
that. She has a strong mind and will and, though deeply emotional,
is not ruled by her emotions, as *Pulsatilla* is for example. However,
when the adrenalin runs out and exhaustion sets in, the person who
needs *Sepia* can become quite worn out and an almost opposite state

is seen: she is burned-out, collapsed, depleted. She will sag and droop mentally and physically. If she can counter this stagnation by activity, she will be able to pick herself up: she is always better for vigorous exercise, dancing or fast walking, and worse for rest, even when exhausted. She is one of those people who is at risk of becoming an exercise fanatic. However, when she gets too weary to exercise then she is completely overcome by exhaustion.

Her mood may range from weepiness and irritability to profound depression. She can be anxious and agitated, wanting to scream or run away from home, leaving her family. She cries when asked questions and is irritable if consoled or sympathized with. She is impatient about everything, especially when contradicted, and she will get extremely irritable when emotional or sexual demands are made on her. She may grow to resent her husband and children and may lash out at them—attacking them verbally, crying for no apparent reason, screaming at them or holding on to things to stop herself from screaming. In these states she is critical, peevish, vexed at the slightest thing, fault-finding, discontented, quarrelsome, nagging, martyred and completely pessimistic.

There is also a less active version of the *Sepia* state in which the person is predominantly silent and moody: she cuts herself off from others, feels uninterested in them and wants to be left alone. She becomes completely indifferent to everyone and everything: she does not care about anything, about her family or loved ones especially, her work, what she looks like, what her house looks like. She says she cannot be bothered; she is worn out, sits and does nothing, for nothing has any meaning. She feels dragged down and miserable and does not want sympathy or consolation. She loses interest completely in all the things with which she was previously happily involved: any activity, people, sex, food, relationships, work. She feels completely flat and cut off from life, empty inside and despairing. She may become suicidally depressed as she feels more and more lost and lonely but is powerless to do anything about it.

She may develop many fears: that she will die soon, that she will become poor and starve, that she will be humiliated. She also fears imaginary evils, ghosts; she even fears thunderstorms though she is energized by watching them. She feels trapped and wants to escape, developing claustrophobia.

Sepia is often needed when women reach their middle years, when their children are much more independent but have not yet left home, when they may feel, yet feel guilty for it, that everyone else in their family has had a chance to develop in life, yet where are they? Suddenly having been a wife and mother does not feel enough—they want their own fulfilment, want to know who they are. They begin to feel resentful of their continuing responsibility to the family, of being trapped.

Sepia is a remedy which is often very strongly indicated at times of hormonal change: puberty, menses, pregnancy, menopause, after an abortion. Often people will say that they have never been well since one of these episodes. *Sepia* subjects have often been more strongly affected by taking a contraceptive pill than others: they may have had headaches, low blood sugar or low energy since being on the Pill. Their emotions are strongly and clearly related to their hormones. It is very highly indicated in so-called post-natal depression.

General and Characteristic Physical Symptoms

- General chilliness, with poor circulation—but subject to hot flushes.
- A general pelvic weakness and lack of tone in the veins and muscles, leading to dragging down, sagging feelings, as if one's insides were about to fall out: prolapse, varicose veins and piles may be particular expressions of this characteristic.
- Problems of menopause including hot flushes, dryness and itching of the vagina.
- A tendency to constipation, backaches and weariness.
- Sensation of a lump or ball in various parts of the body.
- *Sepia* is known as a 'left-sided' remedy—that is, symptoms tend to occur on the left side of the body.
- Sufferers like sour, bitter and tart foods (especially vinegar and pickles), also acid, spicy or highly-seasoned foods; they feel a strong aversion to fats and milk; they crave chocolate.

States and conditions are improved by: violent exercise, dancing, fast walking, occupation.

States and conditions are made worse by: stuffy rooms but also cold air, evening, night, rest, standing or kneeling for long periods, the atmosphere before a storm, sexual intercourse, clothes that are tight around the neck and abdomen.

States and conditions may be caused by: times of hormonal change, hypothyroid conditions, exhaustion.

SILICA

(Silicon dioxide: Quartz, flint, sand)

EMOTIONAL AND PSYCHOLOGICAL CHARACTERISTICS
The *Silica* picture is of someone with a very low level of available energy, even inertia, both physical and mental. These are the kind of people of whom others often unkindly say 'they were born tired.' They are extremely easily fatigued and affected by stress. They are described as lacking grit and stamina, as 'edifices without sand'. They may look quite delicate and fragile, thin and undernourished, indeed they often have been sickly in childhood, children who have failed to thrive.

They are quiet, cautious, timid, unassuming, unaggressive, shy and diffident in manner, never putting themselves forward. However, they are rarely as frail as they look and will usually be found to be quietly strong-willed and determined, even to the point of obstinacy. They are both yielding and obstinate, yielding to others in most cases, but obstinate where anything important is concerned (usually for them a matter of precise fact or principle). They overcome their natural timidity and tendency to anxiety by being very conscientious and working hard so that they do, in fact, achieve quite a lot by dogged persistence and perseverance in whatever they decide to undertake.

They are well aware of not being very strong, of having to ration their energy. They do not do anything that takes too much out of them, living well within their limits and always feeling on the verge of collapse. They go through life avoiding having too many responsibilities because they think they will get overtired and not be able to do what they have undertaken in the conscientious way that suits them. They like to do things they are used to and nothing more. Their deepest fear is that they will not be able to manage all they have to do. They fear breakdown—not a mental breakdown like *Lycopodium*, but a breakdown from exhaustion. They suffer from anticipatory anxiety about the possibility of becoming exhausted. When they do get overtired they often cannot stop overworking for fear of never being able to start again.

Reluctance to undertake anything for fear of failure is the most characteristic *Silica* symptom. Dread of failure and fear of responsibility are greater in this remedy picture than in any other, and it is this fear of failure that underlies their whole lives. Anticipatory anxiety is a major symptom. It shows itself particularly when there is a need to appear in public or to take exams. Their fear is not of failing but of not doing whatever it is as well as it might be done – not of failing exams but of not getting an A. In fact, they usually do well. Their fear comes on long in advance of the event itself, and this distinguishes it from the acute stage fright of *Gelsemium* and *Argentum nitricum*.

If they do decide to undertake some enterprise then they will work very hard and conscientiously and do it well. Their conscientiousness is, in fact, even greater than that of *Arsenicum* because they are not as restless and will stick at things longer. Sometimes they can become ineffective because of their habit of concentrating on very small details, thus losing sight of the big picture. Their fastidiousness and conscientiousness can reach the point of obsession. Their conscientiousness is founded in self-doubt: they think that the only way they will achieve anything at all is to work harder.

Their general low level of self-confidence makes them unassertive: they do not stand up for themselves as a rule and will not defend themselves in an argument or a disagreement. Even though they are intolerant of criticism and contradiction they simply withdraw rather than argue. It is not important for them to succeed in a competition or to dominate another person; it is only important that they do their best. Having said this, they are immovable when it comes to a matter of principle; once they take a stand on anything their obstinacy takes over from their timidity. Their obstinacy nearly always takes the form of resistance or refusal to budge rather than of any onwardly driving energy.

Silica is also one of the main remedies for intellectual burn-out, for those who become truly exhausted from worry or mental effort. They begin not to be able to concentrate well or to focus, their memory gets bad. They lose their train of thought or become distracted, thinking of two things at once, putting their purse in the fridge and the milk in their handbag. This is one of the main remedies for the effects of mental exertion, for intellectual as well as physical fatigue.

It is as well a remedy for many fears: of not being able to carry on, of being away from home, of needles, knives and other sharp or pointed objects (acupuncture, vaccination), of driving, of being robbed, of fear itself. They may be easily discouraged, thinking they are doing the wrong thing, becoming indecisive. They worry over little things, over having got things wrong or even not exactly right.

The *Silica* personality is very self-contained. They like to remain uncommitted in relationships, shying away from closeness and intimacy. They may feel disconnected from others: this is an almost inevitable consequence of their general lack of confidence. Fear of failure also affects their sexual relationships.

Sleep is difficult, especially away from home: there may be terrifying dreams of wrestling with robbers, of murderers, as if about to be throttled; there may be dreams of snakes or dogs. There is a tendency to sleepwalking, especially at times of the new and full moon.

Their nervous systems are generally very sensitive: they are easily startled, jump if touched, cannot work very well if there is a lot of noise or confusion in their environment. They get irritated by trifling things and may fly unexpectedly into a rage at the least noise or irritation once their nervous systems are really shot to pieces.

General and Characteristic Physical Symptoms

- A tendency to thinness.
- Sensitivity to cold and draughts (may wear heavy clothes in summer, and a hat at all times).
- A tendency to repeated colds, possibly developing into respiratory problems.
- Drenching sweats; smelly, sweaty feet. Head sweats that soak the pillow.

- A chronic tendency to suppuration (even the slightest wound suppurates). The person may get a lot of boils, abscesses and bronchial infections.
- There are often sensations of splinters, thorns or needles in the tissues of the skin.
- Brittle nails, covered with white spots.
- Poor appetite; person craves cold food, dislikes hot food, meat, mother's milk; frequently does not assimilate nutrients well from food and may become thin in spite of eating well. Great thirst.

States and conditions are improved by: heat, warm clothing, summer, lying down.

States and conditions are made worse by: cold, draughts, new moon, full moon, before and during thunderstorms, exertion, vaccinations.

States and conditions may be caused by: intellectual strain, vaccination, exposure to cold air, draughts, malnutrition, malabsorption, fright, shock.

STAPHYSAGRIA

(Stavesacre; Larkspur)

EMOTIONAL AND PSYCHOLOGICAL CHARACTERISTICS
When you first meet the person who needs *Staphysagria* he will probably seem to be a nice, kind, gentle person, no trouble to anyone, quiet, pleasant and reserved, perhaps slightly highly-strung. You may wonder whether anyone can be as nice as this man seems to be.

The niceness arises from a long-established habit of not fighting back against any insult, humiliation or attack, of not confronting those who have abused or taken advantage of him. Very occasionally you may get a glimpse of the deep hurt and indignation which have been repressed or suppressed in the past, and some anger may be openly expressed, though it will be quickly suppressed again.

A person needing *Staphysagria* basically controls his feelings when hurt, trying to protect himself from hurt by pretending that nothing has happened and maintaining a dignified front at all costs. This may arise because he has a particularly sensitive nature or constitution, or because of circumstances: it is hard to feel free to show feelings, for instance, in the face of a very stern parent, an overpowering boss, a bullying partner or when part of an oppressed minority.

The capacity to suppress angry and hurt feelings may be turned to good use and the person may become constantly helpful and supportive, seeking to prevent hurt and attack by always being gentle himself, cultivating a kind and peaceable disposition. He may become a little self-righteous and critical, like *Arsenicum*, but he is much less astringent and does not always feel that he is in the right.

If such suppression is a life-long adaptation the man will probably be unconscious of it himself and will genuinely believe himself to be as mild and agreeable as he appears to others. However, eventually this attitude will breed resentment and the well-known silent indignation and reserved displeasure. However well disguised, the underlying state of sensitivity to hurt may eventually be revealed by his attitude of touchiness and over-sensitivity to the slightest thing, he will not be able to keep up being nice for ever. He may easily feel that he is being got at, get upset when people are rude to him, be quick to take offence.

Although he may continue to fail to recognize or to suppress a full expression of anger, he may become easily irritated and excitable, giving way to fits of displaced anger, throwing or breaking things. He will rarely be directly rude, however. When he suppresses his anger he may walk away from the situation, and afterwards feel guilty and be unable to sleep that night. Or he may deflect the anger onto something else, get righteously angry about some just cause.

The need to please everyone eventually saps his confidence and self-esteem. Fears of not being good enough develop, fears of failure, of being unlovable, of being abandoned or hurt. Suppressed anger and resentment may strike deeper and manifest as depression, even suicidal depression with deep feelings of worthlessness. He may turn his unexpressed anger against himself, taking to self-harm.

There are a lot of sexual symptoms in this remedy picture. *Staphysagria* is one of the commonest remedies for sexual obsessions, obsessive sexual fantasies, where sexual thoughts crowd in unasked. There can be insomnia from sexual fantasies. There may be disturbing feelings of increased or uncontrollable sexual desire. On the other hand, decreased sexual passion, impotence and the fear of intimacy are also encountered, as well as sexual problems arising from enforced celibacy. A person may shake, tremble, pass out during sexual intercourse, have flashbacks or anxieties about something that happened in the past. It is a remedy very highly indicated in cases of childhood sexual abuse.

General and Characteristic Physical Symptoms

- Exhaustion, shakiness and trembling from suppressed emotions.
- A loss of voice when angry (the person may become completely unable to speak or make a sound; he opens his mouth to say something and nothing comes out).
- Sighing is characteristic, especially while swallowing.
- There may be acute eruptions of weeping eczema.
- Coughs, headaches, cystitis, stomach ache, toothache, exhaustion may all result from the suppression or delayed expression of anger.
- Wounds, especially the incised wounds of surgery, are painful and slow to heal.
- Sensitive gums (bleeding easily); teeth may be blackened from caries.
- Prey to mosquitoes and other biting insects.
- Symptoms affecting the genito-urinary system: genital warts and tumorous growths, prostatitis, atrophy or induration of the testicles, cystitis, frequency of urination, compulsive masturbation.
- Symptoms connected with menstruation: increased or decreased bleeding, cessation of bleeding (amenorrhoea) after upset, post-menopausal bleeding.
- Great hunger even after eating; the person craves bread, milk and tobacco. Generally thirstless.
- Chilliness; the person wakes in the night feeling cold.

States and conditions are improved by: rest, eating, warmth.

States and conditions are made worse by: exertion, sexual excess, suppressed anger, touch, tobacco, early morning.

States and conditions may be caused by: hypersensitive nature, sexual abuse or assault, humiliation, emotional hurt, oppression, surgery.

STRAMONIUM

(*Datura stramonium; Thorn apple/Jimson weed*)

EMOTIONAL AND PSYCHOLOGICAL CHARACTERISTICS
Stramonium is a plant that has been used for centuries by shamanic healers as a means of penetrating non-ordinary reality – it is what we would call a hallucinogenic substance. Under its influence people have talked with spirits and seen devouring animals, black objects, attacking dogs, elongated faces, images and phantoms, bright and shining objects, and have felt terrified of what they have seen. It can cause wild uncoordinated movements of the body and, in its crude form, has induced madness.

Since substances can cure what they can cause in homoeopathic medicine, this is one of several remedies which in the past were only seen as useful in advanced states of mental illness, mania, hallucination and delirium, where such strong symptoms emerge. Nowadays its action in less intense states is being investigated and it is coming to be used in a wider variety of situations. It is particularly well indicated for a range of anxieties and fears, wild behaviour in children (or adults) and certain types of depression.

The picture of 'crazy' behaviour known from the older *Materia Medica* may still be seen in very distressed children, in hyperactive children, or in acute states of delirium: for example fever, the DTs (delirium tremens), rabies, drug reactions, and of course in people suffering severe states of psychological disorganization.

This state is described as highly agitated, active, driven and possibly violent, with hallucinations, convulsions and constant uncoordinated movements. The person may be restless and raging, very destructive and violent, wanting to fight, bite, take off or tear up her clothes, or smash things; she is incoherently talkative, compulsively shouting and swearing. She suffers enormous fear especially of the dark or shining surfaces, also the fear of being devoured or attacked by animals.

Wherever you see glimpses of this uncontrolled eruption of deep unconscious fears with rage and violence think of *Stramonium*.

This kind of rage and restlessness may be clearly seen in children who have violent tantrums, attack siblings or teddy bears, break toys, stab, who are fascinated by violence or who become obsessed with guns or knives. Destructiveness is a major symptom, accompanied by fear of being destroyed or abandoned. In children you will see sudden outbursts of violence and murderous impulses: they will get absolutely raging mad, but will then settle down again and assume their normal pleasant nature. You may think of it when a child develops superhuman strength during a tantrum, or when a normally mild person gets so angry that she will smash things with more power than you thought she had, getting into a rage to the point of losing control. You may see this behaviour sporadically in adults, but adults have usually been socialized out of it so it is more likely to emerge only in extreme situations.

The anxiety and fear are as strong as that of *Aconite* or *Belladonna*. The major fear is of the dark, with a real terror of being left alone in the dark, at night. Thus *Stramonium* is an important remedy for night terrors: for a child who wakes at night screaming and terrified, not recognizing her parents. She will insist on sleeping with a light on or the curtains open. She has a fear of black things in general, of blackness.

She also experiences a terrible fear of being closed in – severe claustrophobia – a great fear of tunnels and narrow places. There is also a fear of shiny things, of bright and shining objects: mirrors, white things, expanses of water. There are a lot of fears surrounding water (especially running or rushing water), even of having her hair washed. She fears being injured, having an accident, death, dogs. A particular fear of abandonment may be seen in children, especially when they fear being separated from their mother.

You will see these fears clearly manifested in children: they may appear in a more muted form in adults but they will still be there.

Perhaps the affected person will not go on the underground railway systems or down tunnels, will not dare to leave the house. Maybe she will not really give full expression to these fears, but they will be there.

You can imagine using *Stramonium* when you suddenly see another side of a person, a more violent, wilder, more fearful side than you are used to seeing. *Stramonium* presents a picture of the sudden emergence of the repressed shadow side of a person under stress: what has been repressed in this particular case is largely fear and violence (whereas for instance what has been repressed in *Thuja* is sexual material). When such feelings reappear they are completely out of conscious control.

There is also a severe depressive state in this remedy picture: feelings of extreme worthlessness, a sense of being in a garden full of weeds, in a cemetery, alone in a wilderness, abandoned and neglected. The sufferer feels vulnerable to being exposed, to injury, to hurt, even to looking at herself. She has a desire to hide, a fear of mirrors, an aversion to light and a fear of being approached. She seeks to keep herself in shadow.

And, of course, this remedy is still of use in real mental breakdown: acute mania, puerperal mania, delirium tremens. Then the person may speak in tongues, in different languages, in different voices, with great loquacity and laughter. The person may feel as if she has been possessed by a demon, by a devil. She may pick at her bedclothes, expose herself, talk and sing lasciviously.

General and Characteristic Physical Symptoms

- Almost complete absence of pain despite the extreme violence of symptoms.
- Frequently burning thirst but difficulty swallowing water; aversion to all liquids.
- Bright red rash similar to scarlatina.
- Congestive headaches after sunstroke.
- Severe stammering – sufferers will be red in the face until they can get their words out.
- Spasmodic, disorderly, jerky movements; trembling of limbs.
- Twitching of muscles or generalized convulsions; facial contortions.

- Intense fever in delirium; febrile convulsions.
- Frequent cold sweats.

States and conditions are improved by: company, soft light, warmth.

States and conditions are made worse by: dark, night, cold water, glittering objects, being alone, wind.

States and conditions may be caused by: fear, terror, a difficult birth, an operation, a violent rape or attack, a bad trip on drugs, sexual abuse, abandonment (for whatever reason), head injury, rabies, alcoholic intoxication.

SULPHUR

(Brimstone, burning stone)

EMOTIONAL AND PSYCHOLOGICAL CHARACTERISTICS
Sulphur is a difficult remedy to describe adequately because its picture covers such an enormous range of symptoms that any description is bound to leave a lot out. The most common *Sulphur* picture is that of the rather eccentric, untidy person who is not particularly interested in his personal appearance. He often has itchy skin complaints, a lot of red skin and either a florid complexion or red edges to his eyes or mouth. He can be found slumped in a chair endlessly talking and speculating. Traditionally this type has been called the 'ragged philosopher'. Another *Sulphur* type is extremely laid-back, likes the good things in life, is irrepressibly good-humoured and healthy, hospitable and benevolent: the classic *bon viveur*.

One of the major, keynote symptoms of the remedy is that of egocentricity, self-centredness. The person who needs *Sulphur* needs attention and recognition; he makes no apology for wanting to be the centre of attention. When he is on good form this can be very acceptable: a healthy *Sulphur* knows a great deal about a number of subjects, will tell his audience everything he knows, will entertain with all sorts of detailed information about the most surprising things. But he can also become an obsessively self-preoccupied bore who dominates everyone within reach with his latest theories and information, whether they want to hear or not. He has a driving need to be thought well of, to impress intellectually. He thinks relationships are made through imparting knowledge and intellectual argument, but fails to notice his disappearing audience. You can feel very alone with a *Sulphur* personality.

The *Sulphur* type is what is described as 'mentally-identified', the mind is the centre of all operations (regardless of whether the mind is good or not) and emotions are given very little attention. At worst such a person might just ride roughshod over people's emotions, sublimely indifferent to them, genuinely unaware that feelings might be more important than logic.

A person who needs *Sulphur* is characteristically full and over-flowing like a volcano, full of himself, full of ideas, full of plans and theories. Great at initiating things, he rarely finishes them, partly out of his inability to organize the vast amount of information gener-ated, partly out of boredom with details, partly out of laziness. He may have a prodigious memory but has no gift for refining and making selections about what is important and what is not. As long as his energy remains intact and he is achieving and doing well, he remains fine – but he can burn out through overwork and then collapse, often into a deep depression.

Depression is the strongest symptom in this emotional sphere, a deep apathetic depression which looks like extreme laziness to everyone else. *Sulphur* just stops: he does not want to work, or think, or do anything; he just wants to die. He is described as being too lazy to rouse himself and too unhappy to live when he is in this state. Depression also sometimes emerges out of boredom: his restless intellectual energies need a lot of stimulation. With the depression comes an impatience, irritability and moroseness which do not endear him to those who try to help. Weeping often ac-companies the depression.

One of this remedy's main uses might be for teenagers, as when an adolescent falls into a sort of lazy, sullen apathy, losing interest in everything he was interested in before, staying up all hours and then sleeping long into the morning.

Irritability and grumpiness are common features of this remedy picture too, especially in the mornings. The person can be unco-operative, quarrelsome, critical and dissatisfied. He is quick-tempered and irritable, usually over little things; he can at times get carried away and become very bullying and abrasive. But his temper is usually soon over; though he is excitable his mood quickly subsides and he repents his bad temper.

He has a sort of intellectual itchiness and impatience, dislikes slowness and does not suffer fools gladly. He enjoys and is stimulated by argument, argues for argument's sake, and often seems to be looking for a verbal fight. It is as if he cannot be still or fears stillness. He is afraid that this inertia will turn to stagnation and depression or despair. This intellectual restlessness and excitability can make other people feel very dull and insecure in his presence.

Anxiety is strong in the remedy picture: the person may be anxious quite a lot of the time, about what may happen in the future, about his health and the possibility of getting a disease, about a whole range of moral and religious questions which others will feel are completely pointless and unanswerable. 'Who made God?' represents the classic *Sulphur* preoccupation. There can in illness be a quite fussy, picky aspect to him reminiscent of that found in the *Arsenicum* state.

He cannot sleep at night 'on account of the great flow of thoughts' or, once asleep, wakes frequently or becomes wide awake suddenly. He also wakes at 3, 4 or 5 a.m. and sometimes cannot fall asleep again. When he does sleep, it fails to refresh him. He is often drowsy during the day, nodding off in the middle of conversations even, then wakeful at night. He is much better if he takes short sleeps during the day and night.

Underneath the apparent *Sulphur* confidence and bombast there is a great insecurity about how others think of him. The exaggerated display of knowledge and learning, the acquisition and broadcasting of curious information, the personal eccentricities may all be unconsciously directed to attracting approval and recognition, but their effect is all too often to create a barrier between him and others which prevents him from making the relationships he needs.

He may become so completely self-absorbed and indifferent to others that he separates himself from them and lives in a world of his own. He can become paranoid through an exaggerated sense of his own worth.

If he breaks down it may be through becoming alcoholic, and he may even take to the streets, having a lot of the tramp in his make-up. The grandiose ideas which are relatively normal to him may become more serious delusions – for example, he may come to think that the rags he wears are beautiful.

The *Sulphur* picture shows two characteristic polarities of behaviour: a restless, driving omnivorousness, whether for intellectual material or for food and drink, and a contrasting state of complete collapse and disintegration. The person may be out in the world functioning, planning, working successfully or lying late in bed, despairing and drinking.

General and Characteristic Physical Symptoms

- The person is usually warm-blooded, red-faced, uncomfortable in heated rooms or spaces.
- A craving for fresh air, but a dislike of extreme cold.
- Burning sensations and pains, especially burning of the soles of the feet at night and a burning vertex (top of the head).
- Circulation is easily disturbed: sufferers may say that their 'inner thermostat' has stopped working, especially in menopause.
- Dry, rough, scaly skin with a tendency to eruptions, sores and pussy spots. The skin is generally itchy even where there are no eruptions; the person may scratch his skin till it bleeds to get relief.
- Frequent hunger especially around 11 a.m.; the person gets a sinking feeling if he cannot eat. He craves (or dislikes strongly) fat, salt, sweets, spicy foods, pickles. His thirst is marked (especially for water and alcohol).
- Lots of digestive discomfort: diarrhoea which drives him from bed in the early morning; piles.
- Body odour; offensive discharges.

States and conditions are improved by: motion, fresh air.

States and conditions are made worse by: being still (especially standing), heat of the bed, severe cold, washing, 11 a.m., waking, Spring.

States and conditions may be caused by: serious illness, toxic system.

THUJA OCCIDENTALIS

(Arbor vitae, Tree of life, White cedar)

EMOTIONAL AND PSYCHOLOGICAL CHARACTERISTICS
The *Thuja* tree provides wood which is used for making poles and
fences, and it may be useful to keep this in mind when thinking of
the *Thuja* personality – which is one of the most fixed and rigid in
the *Materia Medica*.

What will probably strike you most about people who need *Thuja*
will be their caution and reserve. They will seem friendly enough,
though perhaps a little quiet, but you will never get the sense that
you know them: they protect themselves very carefully. You will only
gradually begin to realize that they have very little self-confidence
and seem to have a constant fear of being 'found out' as bad,
fundamentally unacceptable. They seem to feel guilty, to try to keep
their inner selves secret. They are cautious and mistrustful, secretive,
closed, wary of giving anything away. This is how they appear: they
may consciously have nothing at all to hide, but this attitude has
been part of them since childhood.

They have a sense of being separate from others, which of course
becomes true to some extent because of their secrecy and reserve.
Unconsciously they present to the world an image which does not
quite express what is going on inside: they therefore have a sense of
being double, divided into two parts. They split themselves off from
their feelings and hence lose touch with their sense of self. They feel
that the mind and body are separate, as if the soul is distinct from
the body, that one half of them is separated from the other. They
have fears of going mad, losing control, leaving their bodies; they

feel that something is moving around inside them. They often do not look as if they are happy in their bodies, they can look stiff and solid, wooden: they may feel that their legs are made of wood and that they are brittle like glass, inside. They feel they might break and often look as if they were trying to protect themselves against that possibility.

Depression is strong in the picture (unsurprisingly considering the extent of their suppression of feelings and their deep conviction that there is something wrong and bad about them). They get as stuck in the depression as in everything else, feeling that nothing will ever change. They get tired of life, feeling they have had enough of it, and can become suicidal.

In another mode they are impatient and restive, easily roused to anger. They talk and move hurriedly even though they are not impulsive by nature. They are easily upset by the slightest contradiction or difficulty. They are sensitive and impressionable: music makes them cry.

Psychologically this remedy picture probably covers the greatest range of obsessional symptoms in the *Materia Medica*, even more than those of *Arsenicum* or *Silica*. People who need this remedy have the most fixed ideas, the most rigid thought patterns.

They are very scrupulous over little things and touchy over petty things, too. Their minds are preoccupied with persistent ideas. They get stuck in one track and it is difficult to get them off it. They can be extraordinarily single-minded. When their obsessions get to a pathological level they may become seriously convinced that someone is following them, they may hallucinate that a stranger is sitting beside them, that their body and soul have become separated, that they are made of glass and may break. They may develop fixed ideas that they are under the influence of a superhuman power; they may have delusions and fixed ideas about demons and spirits trying to control their minds. They feel that someone is trying to possess them or trying to manipulate their minds, to make them do things. They fear losing control, going insane.

They are extremely anxious: at the approach of strangers, at how they appear to others; they think something might be in the food, they think they might have cancer or some other illness; they mull over their past failures, feel they have committed a crime, worry about the future, are fearful of their salvation. Sleep is disturbed by anxious, amorous, sometimes frightful dreams, often of falling from a height. There is a tendency to wake at about 3 a.m. and then be unable to get back to sleep.

The people who need this remedy tend to feel ashamed about sexual things, too. They may think it is shameful to have sexual fantasies or to masturbate. The fact of feeling ashamed is the indication for the remedy, the fact that they are secretive about themselves, feeling that they are bad. The origin of these feelings may well be sexual abuse in childhood, and this may indeed often be a major cause of the *Thuja* secretiveness. The splitting off may have become necessary then.

General and Characteristic Physical Symptoms

- Poor physical condition. People who need *Thuja* may look pale, fleshy, with a greasy complexion (perhaps with a yellowish tinge).
- A tendency to retain water; sweatiness.
- The production of excess tissue or mucus or sweat: cysts or styes on the eyelids, warty growths, skin tags, polyps, fibroids, cysts of all sorts.
- Inflammations and discharges from the genital area, usually yellowy-green and offensive. The genital area is sweaty.
- Uncovered parts of the body perspire.
- Complaints tend to favour the left-hand side of the body.
- Arthritis characterized by stiffness and cracking of joints, worse in cold damp weather.
- Asthma is a major symptom.
- Sufferers find it difficult to digest onions or fat; they desire cold drinks, salt, tea; they rarely eat breakfast.
- Tendency to multiple allergies and a weakened immune system.

States and conditions are improved by: cool air, perspiration.

States and conditions are made worse by: exposure to damp cold, heat of the bed, 3 a.m. and 3 p.m., onions, tea, menstruating, the full moon.

States and conditions may be caused by: vaccinations, gonorrhoea or a family history of gonorrhoea, sexual or physical abuse, drinking too much tea.

QUICK KEY TO MAIN SYMPTOMS OF REMEDIES

Remedy	Characteristics	Emotional Conditions	Common Physical Conditions	Improved By	Made Worse By
Acon	fearfulness, shock, mental restlessness, sudden intense onset of symptoms, burning or tingling sensations, severe sensitivity to extreme heat or cold, hypersensitivity	phobias, the after-effects of shock, great fear (death), panic attacks, anxiety, insomnia	hot dry skin, acute fevers, hypertension, palpitations, neuralgia	open air	night, extremes in temperature
Anac	sense of split personality: pleasant/vicious, inferiority complex, cursing or swearing, sensation of a plug or blunt object—of pressure anywhere in the body	lack of confidence, aggressive behaviour, loss of concentration, depression, mood swings, eating disorders	headaches, blistery skin rashes, indigestion, constipation, memory loss	rest, eating	cold, mental exertion, not eating
Arg nit	restlessness, introversion, excitability, impulsiveness, hurriedness, fear of failure,	anxiety, anticipatory or performance anxiety, panic attacks, phobias (esp. claustrophobia)	diarrhoea/wind, sore throat, ulcerations (esp. eye), nervous headache, neurological problems	fresh air	sweat, sugar, heat, deadlines

Remedy	Characteristics	Emotional Conditions	Common Physical Conditions	Improved By	Made Worse By
cont.	sharp, splinter-like sensations, difficulty with co-ordination, sugar cravings				
Arsen album	restlessness (mental and physical), insecurity, the need to control, perfectionism, fault-finding, being overly critical, tidiness, obsessional thoughts, anger, exhaustion that comes on easily, chilliness, thirst for small sips of liquid, burning pains, thin burning discharges	anxiety, phobias, hypochondria, obsessional disorders, insomnia, depression, mood swings, depression, suicidal impulses, self-mutilation, anorexia	asthma, eczema, runny colds, hay fever, haemorrhage, bloody discharges, high blood-pressure, nausea, gastric disturbances, diarrhoea and vomiting	company, heat, exertion	being alone, 12–3 a.m., stuffy rooms, walking, lying down, cold
Aurum	over-conscientiousness, the need to over-achieve, disappointment, being easily offended, aloofness, chilliness, sense of duty, sensitivity to pain, sensations of piercing pain	depression, grief and loss, lack of confid-ence, suicidal thoughts, abusive of alcohol or drugs, quick to anger	bone pain, heart problems (high blood-pressure, angina, palpitations), rheumatism, testicular pain	classical music, summer, fresh air	dark, night, mental exertion

Remedy	Characteristics	Emotional Conditions	Common Physical Conditions	Improved By	Made Worse By
Calc carb	oversensitivity, obstinacy, meticulousness, chilliness, poor circulation, excessive perspiration, weight gain, over-industriousness, lateness in (biological) development, hunger, cravings for eggs or indigestible foods, sour discharges	self-consciousness, depression, anxiety, terrible fears, phobias, eating disorders, insomnia, hyperactivity	glandular problems, fatigue, gallstones, asthma, eczema, rheumatism/arthritis, obesity	warmth and dryness, constipation	injustice, exertion, a full moon, the cold and damp
Gelsem	weariness, collapse, near-paralysis, apprehension, timidity, weakness, heaviness in the limbs, no sense of thirst, tremor	depression, anticipatory anxiety, emotional exhaustion, all sorts of fears, phobias	nervous diarrhoea, nervous headaches, colds and flu, fevers, paralysis or polio, blurred or double vision, post-viral syndrome (ME)	sweating, stimulation	heat, bad news
Ignatia	histrionics, excitability, hypersensitivity, paradoxical symptoms, sighs or yawns, spasms	grief, hysteria, acute anxiety, eating disorders, anger, depression, mood swings, shock, insomnia	spasmodic cough, muscle spasms, trembling, headache (feels like a nail through the head), lump in throat, fleeting pains, constriction in the chest	heat, entertainment, deep breathing	sympathy, 11 a.m., strong smells, cold, worry

Remedy	Characteristics	Emotional Conditions	Common Physical Conditions	Improved By	Made Worse By
Lachesis	histrionics, passionate feelings, suspicion, jealousy, talkativeness, excitability, egoism, vindictiveness, bluish/purplish skin, symptoms on the left side of the body or which move from the left to right side	depression, mood swings, paranoia, persecution anxiety, insomnia, disturbing dreams, alcoholism, phobias	PMS, menopause, high blood-pressure, palpitations, hot flushes, congestive headaches, migraine (on left side), difficulty swallowing, asthma, spontaneous bruising, haemorrhages	discharge, start of period, open air, moderate temperatures	delay in the start of a period (or in getting rid of any discharge), restriction, sleep, sun or heat, being touched on the left side of the body
Lyco	reticence, aloofness, timidity/tyranny, cowardice/arrogance, sentimentality, amorousness, poor muscle tone, chilliness, right-sided or right-to-left symptoms, hunger	lack of self-confidence, performance anxiety, anxiety, phobias, insomnia, flashes of anger, mental confusion, psychosexual problems	indigestion, flatulence, bloating, migraines, bronchitis, pneumonia, psoriasis, catarrh	movement, cool air, occupation	4–8 p.m., waking, heat, contradiction, the pressure of clothing
Nat mur	introversion, reserve, sympathy, sense of living in the past, grudge-holding, crying when alone, sense of responsibility, being easily hurt, craving for salty foods, thirst	extreme grief, depression, eating disorders, anxiety, fatigue, mood swings, fears and phobias, hypochondria, insomnia	PMS, headaches, fluid retention, oily skin, anaemia, constipation, cold sores, hay fever, allergies, asthma, ME	open air, not eating	sympathy, 9–11 a.m., seaside, heat, sun

Remedy	Characteristics	Emotional Conditions	Common Physical Conditions	Improved By	Made Worse By
Nux v	intensity, conscientiousness, perfectionism, abundant nervous energy, liverishness, aggression, impulsiveness, orderliness, over-diligence, touchiness, sensitivity, sympathy, violence, chilliness, shooting pains, hypersensitivity, inertia	anger, irritability, anxiety, depression, exhaustion, hypochondria, suicidal thoughts, insomnia, drug abuse, alcoholism, the after-effects of humiliation or of thwarted ambition	indigestion, constipation, irritable bowel syndrome, allergies, ulcers, muscle spasm, piles, lumbago, high blood-pressure, rhinitis	sleep, heat	waking, 3–4 a.m., contradiction, cold, after meals, stimulants, wind, noise
Phos	hypersensitivity, openness, sentimentality, enthusiasm, affection, impressionability, sympathy, artistic sensibility, burning sensations, craving for cold drinks	apathy, fear, anxiety, alcoholism, depression, mood swings, grief	nosebleeds, haemorrhages, hepatitis/cirrhosis or other liver problems, ulcers, dizziness, hoarseness, kidney degeneration, chest complaints	heat, eating, sleep, massage, touch	cold, electric storms, lying on the left side, dusk
Plat	insecurity, histrionics, sense of split personality, preoccupation with sex, feelings that others are smaller or lower, sensations that the body is bandaged, numbness in parts	fear, eating disorders, anxiety, hysteria, rage, hypochondria, mood swings, suicidal feelings, insomnia, sexual dreams, great sexual desire, jealousy, depression	cramps, numbness, trembling, ovarian pain, haemorrhage in labour, painful periods, vaginitis	open air, eating, sunshine	touch, fasting

Remedy	Characteristics	Emotional Conditions	Common Physical Conditions	Improved By	Made Worse By
Pulsatilla	changeability, dependency, being childlike, crying easily, emotionalism, indecision, mildness, timidity, jealousy, touchiness, chilliness, lack of thirst, bland yellow discharges, craving for ice-cream or pastries	mood swings, fears, panic attacks, agoraphobia, anxiety, hypochondria, silent grief, suicidal thoughts, depression, insomnia, eating disorders	painful periods, colds with catarrh, earache, styes, chilblains, cold in the extremities, varicose veins, heartburn, bloatedness, constipation, measles, eczema	fresh air, sympathy, crying, movement, sitting up, company	hot stuffy rooms, rest, ice-cream, fatty foods, puberty, being alone, evening, lying flat
Sepia	diligence, efficiency, indifference, exhaustion, pessimism, stagnation, sense of a lump or ball in various body parts, left-sided symptoms, hunger, pulsations, oestrogen insufficiency, brownish-yellowish colour to the skin, droopiness	depression, weepiness, apathy, loss of interest in sex, anger, irritability, fatigue, anorexia, 'empty nest' syndrome	poor circulation, dyspepsia, backache, constipation, heavy periods, PMS, menopause, hot flushes, vaginal dryness, pains around the liver, prolapse, varicose veins, bleeding piles	dancing, being alone, vigorous exercise, occupation, sleep, warmth	3–5 p.m., company, being still, sympathy, morning, dusk, hormonal change, cold
Silica	lack of stamina, shyness and insecurity, persistence, stubbornness, conscientiousness, caution, hypersensitivity, easy to startle, slenderness,	lack of self-confidence, fear of failure, fear of breakdown, indecision, anxiety felt long before the event, intellectual	suppuration, respiratory difficulties, recurring colds, sweaty cold feet, abscesses, recurring infections, brittle nails, glandular	heat, wet or humid weather, summer	full moon, new moon, mental exertion, vaccination

Remedy	Characteristics	Emotional Conditions	Common Physical Conditions	Improved By	Made Worse By
cont.	extreme chilliness, splinter-like sensations under the skin, sour perspiration	burnout, difficulty concentrating, irritability, fatigue, insomnia, terrifying dreams	problems, constipation, ME		
Staph	pleasantness, nervousness, reserve, suppressing emotion, touchiness, excitability, tremor, sighs	anxiety, resentment, fits of anger, suppressed grief, indignation, eating disorders, depression, suicidal feelings, after-effects of sexual assault, obsessional sexual ideas	menstrual disturbances, trembling, severe itching, eczema, weeping wounds, effects of cystitis, frequent urination, prostate problems, toothache, caries, styes	rest, eating, warmth	touch, sexual excess, quarrels, humiliation
Stram	aggression, destructiveness, violence, no sensitivity to pain, talkativeness, lack of co-ordination, stammer, aversion to liquids, fear of abandonment	rage, tantrums, agitation, intense fears (of water, tunnels, dogs, dark), panic attacks, night terrors, insomnia, nightmares, hallucinations, depression, mania, behavioural problems, hyperactivity, post-traumatic stress disorder, alcoholism	red skin rash, fevers, delirium, convulsions, muscle twitches, cold sweats, meningitis, whooping cough, DTs, sunstroke, stroke	soft light, company, warmth	dark, being alone, shiny objects, dogs, fright

Remedy	Characteristics	Emotional Conditions	Common Physical Conditions	Improved By	Made Worse By
Sulph	laziness, curiosity, preference for theory over action, self-centredness, discontent, eccentricity/inventiveness, optimism, extroversion, untidiness, red orifices, feeling hot and over-heated (particularly the feet when in bed), burning sensations, irritating discharges, foul-smelling discharges, craving for sugar or sweets, hunger, thirst	intellectual burnout, depression, anxiety, hypochondria, irrita-bility, insomnia, fear of heights, alcoholism, eating disorders	physical complaints that recur, slow recovery, menopause, hypertension, itchy skin eruptions, skin burns, eczema, boils, asthma, allergies, rheumatism, varicose veins, piles, hay fever, diarrhoea at 5 a.m., sleep that is unrefreshing	motion, dry weather, elimination, fresh air	standing, water, bathing, heat of the bed, 11 a.m., sleep, exertion
Thuja	secretiveness, reserve, sense of split personality, rigidity, impatience/hurry, indolence, cold/damp, sweetish perspiration, chilliness, weight gain, left-sided symptoms, thick green discharges, limbs that feel like glass or wood	obsessional thoughts, anxiety, lack of self-confidence, depression, suicidal feelings, insomnia, sexual guilt, paranoia, impatience, hypochondria, hallucinations	fluid retention, genital warts, asthma, arthritis, allergies, rheumatism, obesity, deformed nails, headaches, new growths, catarrh, vaginal dis-charge, dry hair/dandruff, neuralgia, ovarian pain (left-sided), chronic urinary infections	heat, perspiring, motion	3 a.m./3 p.m., wet weather, vaccinations, onions, tea, contradiction

Appendix One

———

FURTHER READING

Silvano Arieti, *Understanding and Helping the Schizophrenic: A Guide for Family and Friends* (Basic Books, 1979)

Ellen Bass and Laura Davis, *The Courage to Heal* (Harper & Row, 1988)

Peter Chappell, *Emotional Healing with Homoeopathy* (Element Books, 1994)

Kim Chernin, *The Hungry Self: Women, Eating and Identity* (Virago, 1985)

Catherine Coulter, *Portraits of Homoeopathic Medicines* (3 vols; Berkeley, CA: North Atlantic Books, 1987–89)

Luis Detinis, *Mental Symptoms in Homoeopathy* (Beaconsfield Publishers, 1994)

Piero Ferrucci, *What We May Be* (Thorsons, 1992)

Douglas M. Gibson, *Studies of Homoeopathic Remedies* (Beaconsfield Publishers, 1987)

Eliana Gill, *Outgrowing the Pain: A Book for and about Adults Abused as Children* (Bantam, 1983)

Richard Gillett, *Overcoming Depression: A Practical Self-help Guide* (Dorling-Kindersley, 1987)

Rima Handley, *Homoeopathy for Women* (Thorsons, 1993)

Judith Lewis Herman, *Trauma and Recovery* (Pandora, 1992)

Sandra Horn, *Coping with Bereavement: Coming to Terms with a Sense of Loss* (Thorsons, 1989)

Jacques Jouanny, *The Essentials of Homoeopathic Materia Medica* (Boiron, France, 1984)

Alice Miller, *Banished Knowledge* (Virago, 1990)

Robin Murphy, *Fundamentals of Materia Medica*, vols i & ii (privately published, 1988)

Elisabeth Kubler-Ross, *On Death and Dying* (Macmillan, 1970)

Linda Sanford, *Strong at the Broken Places: Overcoming the Trauma of Childhood Abuse* (Virago, 1991)

Shirley Trickett, *Coming Off Tranquillizers and Sleeping Pills* (Thorsons, 1991)

Appendix Two

USEFUL ADDRESSES
AND TRAINING COURSES

UK

Society of Homoeopaths
2, Artisan Road
Northampton NN1 4HU
Tel: 01604 21400

US

Homoeopathic Education Services
2124 Kitteredge Street
Berkeley, CA 94704

North American Society of Homoeopaths
c/o Valerie O'Hanlan
4712 Aldrich Avenue
Minneapolis, MN 55409

AUSTRALIA

Society of Classical Homeopathy
2nd Floor
Paxton House
90, Pitt Street
Sydney 2000

NEW ZEALAND

New Zealand Institute of Classical Homeopathy
c/o Gwynneth Gibson
24 Westhaven Drive
Tawa, Wellington

SOUTH AFRICA

Joyce Bagnall
c/o A. G. Bagnall
PO Box 3179
Durban 400
Natal

Homoeopathic Pharmacies and Suppliers

In the UK you will be able to buy most of the remedies mentioned in this book in low potencies from local pharmacies or health food stores. If you have any difficulty, you can order very high-quality remedies by phone or post from:

Helios
97 Camden Road
Tunbridge Wells
Kent TN1 2QP
Tel: 01892 537254

Remedies are also available from:

Ainsworths
38 New Cavendish Street
London W1M 7LH

Weleda UK Ltd
Heanor Road
Ilkeston
Derbyshire DE7 8DR

Bottles, boxes and envelopes for storing remedies can be obtained from:

The Homoeopathic Supply Company
4, Nelson Road
Sherringham
Norfolk NR26 8BU

Training Courses

If you wish to train to practise homoeopathic medicine then apply to one of the following Colleges for details of their courses:

The British School of Homoeopathy
23 Sarum Avenue
Melksham
Wiltshire SN12 6BN

The College of Classical Homoeopathy
Othergates Clinic
45 Barrington Street
Tiverton
Devon EX16 6QP

The College of Homoeopathy
Regent's College
Inner Circle
London NW1 4NS

The London College of Classical Homoeopathy
Morley College
61 Westminster Bridge Road
London SE1 7HT

The Northern College of Homoeopathic Medicine
Swinburne House
Swinburne Street
Gateshead
Tyne & Wear NE8 1AX

The North West College of Homoeopathy
23 Wilbraham Road
Fallowfield
Manchester M14 6FB

The School of Homoeopathy
Yondercott House
Uffculme
Devon EX15 3DR

INDEX

Including Index of Symptoms and Remedies

This index serves a dual purpose, acting as both book index and symptom index or repertory.

To find where a specific topic is discussed in the book refer to the pages cited after that named topic in the index.

To find out which remedy pictures include specific emotional and psychological symptoms refer to the remedies cited after that named symptom in the index. If a symptom is followed by the name of a remedy then that symptom is part of that remedy picture and will be found in the *Materia medica* description of that remedy.